PSYCHIATRY, GENETICS
AND PATHOGRAPHY

Psychiatry, Genetics
and
Pathography

A TRIBUTE TO ELIOT SLATER

Editors

MARTIN ROTH

VALERIE COWIE

Assisted by
BRIAN BARRACLOUGH

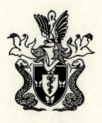

GASKELL PRESS

LONDON

1979

The Gaskell Press is the imprint of the Royal College of Psychiatrists
17 Belgrave Square, London (SW1X 8PG)

© *The Royal College of Psychiatrists 1979*

British Library Cataloguing in Publication Data

   Psychiatry, genetics and pathography
1. Psychiatry—Addresses, essays, lectures
I. Roth, Martin   II. Cowie, Valerie   III. Slater, Eliot
   616.8′9   RC458

ISBN 0 902241 05 2

Printed in Great Britain by Headley Brothers Ltd The Invicta Press Ashford Kent and London

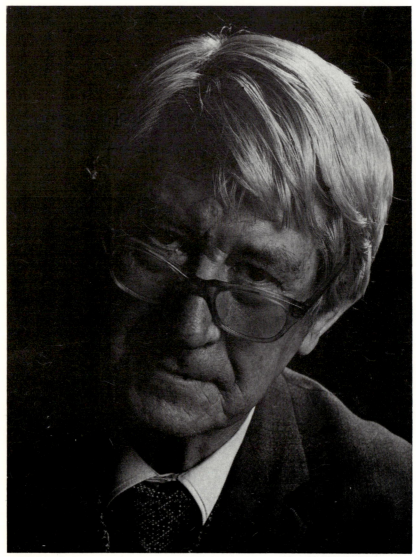

Photograph by RICHARD LEVIN, OBE, RDI

Eliot Trevor Oakeshott Slater

CBE MA MD (Cantab) FRCP FRC Psych HonLLD (Dundee)

Born, 28 August 1904; son of Gilbert Slater, MA, DSc and Violet Slater (née Oakeshott)
Educated at Leighton Park, University of Cambridge, and St George's Hospital, London

Medical Officer, Maudsley Hospital, 1931–39; Rockefeller Foundation Fellowship for study in Munich and Berlin, 1934–35; Medical Research Council research grant, 1935–37; Gaskell Gold Medallist in Psychiatry, 1938; Clinical Director, Sutton Emergency Hospital, 1939–45; Physician in Psychological Medicine, National Hospital, Queen Square, London, 1946–64; Member of the Royal Commission on Capital Punishment, 1949; Senior Lecturer, Institute of Psychiatry, University of London, 1950–59; President, Section of Psychiatry, Royal Society of Medicine, 1958–59; Director, Medical Research Council Psychiatric Genetics Unit, Maudsley Hospital, 1959–69; Litchfield Lecture, Oxford University, 1959; Galton Lecture, 1960; Maudsley Lecture, 1960; Editor-in-chief, *British Journal of Psychiatry*, 1961–72; Honorary Lecturer, Institute of Psychiatry, 1966–71; Geoffrey Vickers Lecture; Mental Health Trust, 1973; Theodosius Dobzhansky Memorial Award, 1978.

Fellow Eugenics Society
Honorary Fellow American Psychiatric Association
Ehrenmitglied der Deutschen Gesellschaft für Psychiatrie und Nervenheilkunde
Honorary Fellow Royal Society Medicine
Honorary Fellow Royal College of Psychiatrists

Books: *Introduction to Physical Methods of Treatment in Psychiatry* (with W. Sargant), 1944; *Patterns of Marriage* (with M. Woodside), 1951; *Psychotic and Neurotic Illnesses in Twins*, 1953; *Clinical Psychiatry* (with W. Mayer-Gross and M. Roth), 1954; *Delinquency in Girls* (with J. Cowie and V. Cowie), 1968; *The Genetics of Mental Disorders* (with V. Cowie), 1971.

Exhibition of paintings at the Loggia Gallery, London, 1977

CONTRIBUTORS

German Berrios
Lecturer, University of Cambridge

Desmond Curran
Emeritus Professor of Psychiatry, University of London

Kenneth Davison
Honorary Lecturer in Psychiatry,
University of Newcastle upon Tyne

W. Edwards Deming
Consultant in Statistical Studies,
Washington, USA

Lindon Eaves
Lecturer in Psychology,
University of Birmingham

Erik Essen-Möller
Emeritus Professor of Psychiatry,
University of Lund, Sweden

G. Ettlinger
Professor of Neuropsychology,
Institute of Psychiatry, London

Hans Eysenck
Professor of Psychology,
Institute of Psychiatry, London

Irving I. Gottesman
Professor of Psychology,
University of Minnesota, USA

Edward Hare
Physician,
The Bethlem Royal and Maudsley Hospitals, London

Leonard L. Heston
Professor of Psychiatry,
University of Minnesota, USA

Einar Kringlen
Professor of Psychiatry,
University of Oslo, Norway

Denis Leigh
Physician,
The Bethlem and Maudsley Royal Hospitals, London

César Pérez de Francisco
Professor of Psychiatry,
University of Mexico

P. Polonio
Professor of Psychiatry,
University of Lisbon, Portugal

David Rosenthal
Chief Laboratory of Psychology, National Institute of Mental Health,
Bethesda, Maryland, USA

Martin Roth
Professor of Psychiatry,
University of Cambridge

The late James Shields
Former Reader in Psychiatric Genetics
Institute of Psychiatry, London

Eliot Slater
Honorary Consulting Psychiatrist,
The Bethlem and Maudsley Royal Hospitals, London

Patrick Slater
Senior Lecturer in Mathematical Psychology,
St George's Hospital Medical School, London

I. A. Syed
Formerly Research Assistant in Psychology,
Institute of Psychiatry,
London

Sedat Topçu
Lecturer in Social Psychology,
Ankara University, Turkey

Moya Woodside
Research Psychiatric Social Worker,
Andrew Duncan Clinic,
Edinburgh

CONTENTS

Foreword by Sir Martin Roth

SOCIAL PSYCHIATRY

EPILEPSY

METHODOLOGY

PERSONAL IMPRESSIONS

APPENDIX

FOREWORD

In this tribute in his seventy-fifth year by a number of his colleagues, friends and contemporaries, the contributions have come mainly from those who have been associated with one or other of the central interests of his professional life: psychiatric genetics and clinical psychiatry.

But this tribute also celebrates one more stage in the life of a man of rare intellectual vigour and passion. As his recent publications, including those we have chosen to include in this volume, testify, the creative phase of his life continues and although the emphasis in his intellectual activities is not where it was a decade ago there is no break in the continuity of his quest for knowledge and understanding. These two, understanding (in the sense of Jaspers) and knowledge, have always been naturally reconciled in him. Although painstaking to the most minute particular in his scientific work he was never tormented with doubt in the manner of some men of scientific spirit faced with the patchy uncertainties of clinical evidence. It was intuition and experience that made him bold and crisp in clinical formulation.

In the insights that permeate his paintings the same features are evident. A walk round an exhibition of his pictures also shows the familiar search behind the appearances for an order that may be approached but lies beyond reach. He has enrolled for a Ph.D. in Shakespearean studies in the seventy-third year of his life. The sensibility and deep compassion of the first essay on the Sonnets of Shakespeare that so surprised some people will be harnessed with his gifts as a mathematician to undertake the literary and linguistic analysis needed. It is recognizably the same man, the same voyage of discovery as in the scientific papers and the autobiographical passages of *Man, Mind and Heredity*.

In the years that have elapsed since that work brought Slater's most important scientific papers together within the pages of a single volume his contributions have come into sharper focus. He is best known in the world of psychiatry and medicine for his investigations into the genetics of schizophrenia, manic-depressive illness and the neurotic constitution and for the emphasis he laid on the importance of the biological disciplines for the advancement of scientific knowledge of mental disorder. But placed in their historical context his contributions acquire a wider significance.

Eliot Slater was the first British psychiatrist of the modern era who had natural mathematical gifts and received a rigorous training as a biological scientist. Early in his career he came under the influence of R. A. Fisher and began to apply modern statistical methods to the solution of problems in clinical psychiatry. His first papers on the inheritance of manic-depressive psychosis set new standards of rigour, clarity and assurance in the handling of evidence. They were published before the appearance of Bradford Hill's *Principles of Medical Statistics* which familiarized a generation of medical scientists with the numerical methods that stemmed from Fisher's discoveries.

It is the logic of statistical method rather than that of any one or other laboratory discipline that constitutes the central and most characteristic feature of modern clinical science. The wide dissemination of the work of Fisher and the bio-statisticians who followed him, and the use of tests of significance to evaluate the results of investigation, was a distinctive feature which for many decades distinguished clinical science in Great Britain from that of other countries.

The disparity was particularly striking in psychiatry and for similar reasons. A number of able men began to apply measurements as precise as the situation would permit and to use statistical methods in the analysis of findings. Lionel Penrose brought his talents to bear on the problems of subnormality and the measurement of intelligence. His classical work related to these matters rather than to questions of clinical psychiatry and psychiatric diagnosis.

However, British psychiatry was fortunate in having a youthful pioneer in the use of the new statistical methods, who also received a thorough grounding in clinical psychiatry. It was a stroke of fortune that Eliot Slater was selected for training in genetics and psychiatry in Munich. Since the publications of his early thirties to the present day he has handled data with a dexterity, an inventiveness and an elegance in reasoning and analysis that have probably not been equalled by any other psychiatric investigator. This remains true today despite the fact that the versatility and power of statistical methods has advanced in recent years.

It was through the force of his example more than any other influence that clinical research in psychiatry in Great Britain acquired its high repute and its most distinctive features. Although the gap has narrowed in the last fifteen to twenty years and has vanished in some places, the disparity in styles of enquiry and in scholarship remains in any comparison between Great Britain and other European countries, with the exception of Scandinavia.

Slater urged the application of biological science to psychiatric problems, and favoured the use of precise measures but he has always retained a profound respect for clinical observation as the central skill of the psychiatrist. In this connection the paper by James Shields raises some points of general importance in addition to shedding light on Slater's diagnostic practice. Slater used neither behaviour rating scales nor estimates of inter-observer reliability. In his genetical studies, for example, he made the psychiatric diagnosis of both twins and he alone decided whether the pair was monozygotic or dizygotic. As he put it in *Man, Mind and Heredity,* 'These were the days before anyone thought of double-blind diagnoses, and the only way to scientific integrity was to set the standards of evidence for a firm diagnosis, and for a "probable" diagnosis, and try to abide by them consistently, even when one saw the evidence going against the working hypothesis'. Yet, as Shields points out, a number of positive findings in the clinical genetic studies of Slater and his colleagues could be shown not to have stemmed from the diagnostician's knowledge of the diagnosis made of the illness in a close relative. For it was possible to exclude any contribution from this source of bias.

There is much in these comments to give the modern psychiatric investigator food for thought. The view that in psychiatric research valuable results are most likely to accrue when clinical diagnostic judgements are excluded in favour of 'objective' measures misconceives the situation. The diagnostic schemes the psychiatric investigator brings to bear in the study of clinical phenomena are an indispensable precondition for the gathering of relevant and worthwhile observations. If he uses his nosological concepts with skill and intelligence they will serve him to differentiate figure from background; without them much of what he records is likely to be noise. Rating scales have their place and their value as a complement to a psychiatric assessment and diagnosis. But they lack the flexibility and analytic power of a range of descriptive schemas. To jettison the latter is to throw the baby out with the bathwater.

Those inclined to dismiss methods Slater employed during the greater part of his professional life as outmoded need to be reminded that almost the entire corpus of knowledge we possess about the diagnosis, heredity, aetiology and treatment of psychiatric disorders has originated from clinical observations undertaken by the same methods. Now traditional phenomenological psychiatry is not lacking in blind spots. Its categories and dichotomies may have been over-simple. But they made for hypotheses that were crisp, risky and refutable.

However, if diagnostic concepts are hypotheses those who use them must be alert to the evidence which refutes or modifies them. Otherwise diagnoses ossify into dogmas that obstruct progress. Shields provides several examples of refutations recognized by Slater. The fact that it is through such refutations that progress is made does not have to be emphasized nowadays. One of the most interesting refutations is to be found in the studies by Slater and his colleagues of the schizophrenia-like psychoses of epilepsy in 1963. Here the hypothesis that a specific genetical factor was a necessary precondition for the development of a schizophrenic syndrome was refuted by the finding that the psychoses that had temporal lobe lesions underlying them were devoid of genetical cause.

Several papers in the section 'Psychiatric Genetics' place on record new observations in fields of investigation in which Slater has been active in the past. Reference has been already made to Shields's objective and illuminating analysis of Slater's diagnostic methods. His sudden death shortly before the publication of this volume interrupted a partnership with Eliot Slater that extended over more than thirty years. It creates a gap in the British psychiatric scene that will prove difficult to repair. Shields was able to carry out a final revision of his own paper and to make some emendations in the joint paper with Gottesman only a few weeks before his death. It seems fitting that the first of his posthumous publications should appear in a volume dedicated to Eliot Slater. In the remaining papers in this section Gottesman and Shields give more precise definition to the schizoid phenotype, Rosenthal discusses the problems of investigating the heredity of behavioural disorders and Polonio gives a brief account of a clinical investigation of a large material of affective cases. Essen-Möller describes the concepts of 'continuity' and discontinuity that stem from the teaching of Sjöbring. This advances a theory of a neurotic constitution similar in certain respects to that formulated in the classical paper of 1944 by Eliot and Patrick Slater. In this volume Patrick Slater, who has collaborated with his brother in several enquiries, contributes a paper on repertory grid techniques, which he has done a great deal to define, and a theoretical study of aggression in a joint contribution with Syed and Topçu.

Eysenck and Eaves examine the contribution of hereditary factors to social attitudes. W. Edwards Deming shows the way towards the development of economic screening tests with a high yield of positives in the course of psychiatric surveys. Edward Hare, in a provocative paper, proposes means whereby psychiatry might be relieved of some of its growing burden of anxieties of social origin. Ettlinger describes some studies in experimental epilepsy stimulated in part by Slater's observations on the association between temporal lobe epilepsy and psychoses. Berrios's paper in the same section traces the development of ideas regarding the relationship between epilepsy and psychosis in nineteenth-century France and shows that many questions which exercise contemporary psychiatrists in this difficult territory were adumbrated by the clinical perceptions of many psychiatrists of the last century.

In the section on pathography there is an important new paper on Edvard Munch by Einar Kringlen. Denis Leigh's contribution has the same title as Mannheim's and Slater's paper of 1947 in the *British Journal of Medical Psychology*. It is a particular pleasure to publish two new papers by Eliot Slater himself. The paper on the creative personality is one of the fruits of his joint enquiries with Alfred Meyer into the personality of musical men of genius. The essay on Hamlet is especially valuable for the insight it provides into those aspects of Slater's creative work that would be unfamiliar to those who have read only his scientific publications. He employs a scholar's knowledge of Shakespeare's plays and a constant aware-ness of detail to advance hypotheses that are tested with a simplicity and elegance that appeal to the poet. His inner eye and empathy enable him to develop an original notion into a rich, suggestive and fertile exercise in psychopathological exploration. His 'frivolous piece' is written with a delicacy of feeling for language that makes a memorable contribution to Shakespearean scholarship. The trenchant critic of psychoanalysis as science advances his own psychodynamic theory for a piece of detective work. No one knows, or can ever know, what was in Shakespeare's mind. But at the end the case has been made that it could well have happened thus.

Happily, contributions continue to flow from Slater's pen. There have been a number of recent papers in journals of Shakespearean scholarship. During the last decade he has tilted against the blind arrogance that sacrifices the beauties of nature and wild life to trivial and meretricious objectives. He has written eloquently in favour of voluntary euthanasia. His recent reviews range from books on the abuse of psychiatry in the Soviet Union to philosophical work on memory and mind, which show him sifting fact from fantasy and confusion, with a sharpness and penetration seemingly unaltered over fifty years.

His interest in the spiritual and speculative life has recently led him to read Jung. His outlook appears to find room for both the austere empiricism of Popper and Jung's mysticism. Whether these are for him universes apart or philosophies with some ground in common will doubtless emerge from future writing that readers of his Mapother Lectures will await with keen anticipation.

This book is a tribute and a celebration. It celebrates the life of a man whose many-sided contributions have enriched the scientific study of mental life and whose generosity and nobility of spirit seem inseparable from his achievement.

MARTIN ROTH

PSYCHIATRIC GENETICS

SCHIZOID PHENOTYPES IN THE CO-TWINS OF SCHIZOPHRENICS

THE SIGNALS AND THE NOISES

I. I. Gottesman, J. Shields and L. L. Heston

Theories which combine correct and false facts are more dangerous to science than complete errors; and hypotheses which are only 'justified in a certain sense' always create confusion because the necessary reservations cannot always be stated. Clearcut concepts can only be formed if we ruthlessly reject everything that does not belong to them, regardless of whether we are dealing with simple problems or with entire theories.

Eugen Bleuler (1950, p 465)

We learn more by noting which of the traits are much more, or less, common in one group than in either of the others. Put in this way, the abnormal personalities of the schizophrenic group are more frequently paranoid, anergic, eccentric or lacking in feeling, and are less frequently diagnosed as emotionally labile or alcoholic than are psychopaths in other kinds of family . . . All these are descriptions by friends and relatives of actual people and from them a vague picture emerges which is very much that which clinicians describe as 'schizoid'. The same or similar words or phrases occur in descriptions of abnormal personalities from the other families, but much less frequently, not in such concentrated form, and they are usually submerged by descriptions of a very different tone.

Eliot Slater (1953, pp 82-3)

Bleuler's admirable strictures and logical criterion for a concept were contained in a footnote in his 1911 classic. Would that we could adhere to them in 1977. The identification of a reliable clinical phenotype (exophenotype) is paramount to further progress in discovering the aetiology of schizophrenia since behavioural-genetic analysis requires such an indicator, one

---

The ideas in this paper have evolved over time in the spirit of self-correction exemplified by our mentor Eliot Slater. Considerable overlap occurs with two previously published papers, Shields, Heston and Gottesman (1975) and Gottesman, Shields and Heston (1976). The two American authors (IIG and LLH) were attached to Slater's MRC Psychiatric Genetics Unit as Visiting Workers in 1963 and 1965 respectively and have been 'attached' to him since.

without surplus meaning. Schizoidia or schizoid personality has been considered such an indicator since 1909 (according to Essen-Möller, 1946) when Gadelius commented on the unreasonableness and inaccessibility to argument that he saw in relatives of schizo-phrenics; he labelled such traits 'pre-catatonic'. Although Kretschmer's theories (since 1921) popularized the idea of a schizoid dimension continuous with normal personality but differing quan-titatively, the term schizoid probably orginated in E. Bleuler's clinic. Kahn, an assistant to Kraepelin, used the term in 1921 (cf. Essen Möller, 1946); his 1923 study on the offspring of dual-mating schizophrenics (*The Schizoid and Schizophrenia in Heredity*) aimed to elucidate the two separate genetic components that he posited as necessary for the development of schizophrenia—one for schizo-phrenic psychosis and one for schizoidia. The problems of defini-tion he faced are with us today but it is little consolation that we have the insight. Slater's observations (above) coming from a clinician with genetic knowledge, have inspired us to take a fresh look at the problem.

Given the justifiable interest in the concept of schizoidia, how would we ever know when we had an indicator of it that Bleuler might have accepted as 'clearcut'? It would have to be reliably measured and independent of the state or stage of the schizo-phrenic process itself (ideally, it could be determined prenatally, but then we would have left the realm of *psycho*pathology). It should be distributed differently in schizophrenics compared to persons with other psychiatric disorders and compared to members of the general population unrelated to patients (cf. Meehl and Rosen, 1955). The next step would be to carry out family and twin studies to see whether in fact the concept as defined could be used as a genetic marker of the predisposition to schizophrenia. A good genetic marker would be present in the identical co-twins of probands whether the latter were unaffected, affected, or in remission (*pace* genetic heterogeneity *pro tempore*). It should occur to a much lesser extent in fraternal co-twins and siblings and other relatives in a way to conform to some genetic hypothesis. Further barriers to the detection of a good indicator of schizoidia arise because of the dynamic nature of both personality and of genes; thus it may require a certain stage of development or an ethical stressor to reveal a phenotype relevant to the genotype of interest, schizo-phrenia (cf Gottesman, 1974).

When the record-keeping manuals for psychiatric taxonomy are consulted (on both sides of the Atlantic) the following phrases recur in connection with the glossary definition of schizoid personality: excessive shyness, excessive reserve, conspicuous aloofness, notably introspective, and eccentricity of conduct. On the face of it such a list suggests some kind of precision in the description of a personality type that may be at a greatly increased risk for developing schizophrenia. Recalling that the lifetime risk for the latter is close to 1 per cent of the general population surviving to age 55 (Slater and Cowie, 1971), the fallibility of the descriptors as predictors becomes apparent too soon. For example, the work of MacFarlane, Allen and Honzik (1962) with the behaviour problems seen in *normal* children observed over a 14-year period in Berkeley, California, reports the following peak prevalences of traits selected by us for their overlap with the phrases above from the world of psychiatry:

Excessive reserve —59% of 10-year-old girls, 52% of 11-year-old boys

Excessive shyness—37% of 11-year-old girls, 22% of 12-year-old boys

Oversensitiveness—53% of 6-year-old girls, 59% of 10-year-old boys.

Sombreness —33% of 6-year-old girls, 36% of 5-year-old boys.

Singling out the trait of oversensitiveness, the authors comment that it was like the common cold, almost everybody had it (p 114). The conclusion is obvious: traits with such high base rates are useless in predicting an event that has a risk in the general population of 1 per cent. The data on normal children make the data from the follow-up studies of shy, withdrawn children seen as patients in child guidance clinics less surprising. Morris *et al*, (1954) and Michael *et al*, (1957) found very few of such child patients grew up to be schizophrenic adults.

Given this latitude in the use of schizoidia, it is worth noting that investigators since Kahn differed widely in their reports of the prevalence of schizoid personality among relatives of schizophrenics. The rates for schizoid personality and schizophrenia in sibs of probands, respectively, were calculated as 3.6 per cent and 11.5 per cent by Luxenburger (1936) and as 31.5 per cent and 14.3 per cent by Kallmann (1938) (see Zerbin-Rüdin, 1967, p 499).

However, it is very important to distinguish between the prediction problem in the general population and the one within the family of a schizophrenic proband. The point is made by Shields *et al* (1975) with respect to Huntington's chorea.

> Let us assume that several children of parents with Huntington's disease are observed to be fidgety and that it is hypothesized that they are the carriers of the abnormal gene. It is predicted that the fidgety children *in Huntington families* will develop Huntington's chorea and that their siblings will not, but it is not predicted that all fidgety children in the general population are at risk for Huntington's disease. To the extent that fidgetiness is a common

characteristic of children, the indicator will be an imperfect one. Some
children of Huntington's patients may be fidgety for reasons other than the
specific Huntington gene . . . It makes sense to us to see whether a high risk
hypothesis, genetic or environmental, works in schizophrenic families without arguing that it must work equally well in the general population.

It is our contention that not all theories about the aetiology of
schizophrenia are equally meritorious. As clinicians with a genetic
bent and a Popperian conscience, we believe that the theories
should be pushed to their limits and hazarded to refutation, or, at
the least, made ready for testing. We are enthusiastic about, but not
committed to, two different genetic theories each of which provides
for important contributions from the environment broadly defined
(Gottesman and Shields, 1967, 1972; Heston, 1970; Shields, 1971;
Shields, Heston and Gottesman, 1975; Slater, 1958; Slater and
Cowie, 1971). The balance of this paper shows the result of con-
frontation and compromise between polygenic and monogenic
orientations towards the aetiology of schizophrenia in the service of
testability and refutation. Although we confidently expect our
brethren in the fields of molecular biology and developmental genetics to administer the *coup de grâce* to the hydra-headed schizophrenia problem, their strategies will proceed most efficiently with
guidance from psychiatric geneticist experienced in twin and family
studies (cf Shields and Gottesman, 1973).

Semantic Confusion versus Semantic Clarification

Semantic and logical problems have plagued the concept of
schizoidia from the beginning. Most troublesome has been the
extent to which the concept implies a phenotypic resemblance to
schizophrenia,* or a genotypic connection with it, or as Essen-
Möller (1946) believed, both.

We shall differentiate and define four uses of the term schizoid,
three of which have no aetiological implications:

Sd 1—Schizoid in the literal sense of resembling schizophrenia
phenotypically but in a diluted fashion. This is how the word
is used in the accepted diagnostic term *schizoid personality*,
meaning shy, sensitive, aloof or eccentric (American
Psychiatric Association, 1968; General Register Office, 1968).
It does *not* imply a genealogical or aetiological connection

---

*It is in this sense that the concept has attracted the most attention. Scholarly reviews by
Essen-Möller (1946) and by Planansky (1972) delineate much of the background against
which our views should be considered. Despite the criticisms we level at the concept
throughout this paper, we would not deny the heuristic value already proved for the term
schizoid as a powerful explanatory variable in the hands of some investigators for some
kinds of research closely related to our interests (e.g. / Ødegaard, 1946, and Stevens, 1969).

with schizophrenia. It shades into the normal. It can be extended to include paranoid personality. Though not standard usage, it could also be extended to cover persons such as those with a *T* score over 70 on the Schizophrenia scale of the MMPI or who score highly on a test of thought disorder that differentiates schizophrenics from others. It would not include depressives, criminals or the mentally retarded since they cannot generally be described as schizophrenic-like.

Sd 2—Psychiatric disorders occurring in the families (usually the twins or first degree relatives) of schizophrenics, *whether resembling schizophrenia or not,* and whether or not they occur more frequently in schizophrenia than control families. A genetic connection with schizophrenia is not implied. (These are the potential or eligible components for Heston's (1970) 'schizoid disease'.)

Sd 3—Disorders, whether occurring in a person who is the relative of a schizophrenic or not, that belong to a class found more often in the families of schizophrenics than in their controls, (These are akin to the 'schizophrenia spectrum disorders' of Rosenthal and Kety's group, including those of the 'extended' spectrum (Kety *et al* 1975; Rosenthal 1975).)

Sd 4—A diagnosis or behavioural trait or combination of traits, whether diagnosable as abnormal or not, which is believed to indicate either a probable carrier of the schizophrenic gene (monogenic hypothesis) or a high risk genotype (polygenic hypothesis). This usage resembles the schizotype of Rado (1962) and Meehl (1962), including the compensated schizotype, but is not necessarily wedded to Meehl's (1964, 1973) checklist of schizotypic signs or to a monogenic hypothesis.

Rather than arbitrarily modify the meaning of terms used by the DSM II, Heston, Rosenthal or Meehl, we shall refer to these uses of the term schizoid as *Sd 1, Sd 2, Sd 3,* and *Sd 4* respectively. *Sd 1, 2* and *3* overlap to an extent that cannot be determined until much more extensive epidemiological and family investigation has been carried out using *Sd 1* and *Sd 3* as index cases.

We shall illustrate the overlap of *Sd 1, 2* and *3* schematically in a Venn diagram. Let us start with persons in a population who have *Sd 3* conditions. They are represented in Figure 1a by a circle with broken outline. These, then, are people with disorders of a kind found to occur more frequently in the relatives of schizophrenics than in controls. According to Kety *et al* (1968) they would include criminals, and according to Heston (1966) some mentally retarded. Of course, which disorders are identified as *Sd 3* will differ from study to study, and their prevalence will differ from population to

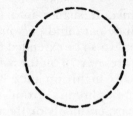

(a) Persons with *Sd 3* conditions

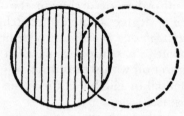

(b) Persons with *Sd 3* conditions (broken outline) plus *Sd 1* (vertical hatching)

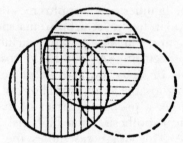

(c) Persons with *Sd 3* conditions (broken outline) plus *Sd 1* (vertical hatching) plus *Sd 2* (horizontal hatchings)

Fig. 1. Schematic of relationship between *Sd 1, 2, and 3*.

population. How far they may be related to schizophrenia genetically (*Sd 4*) is another matter.

Sd 1, according to our terminology, means 'resembling schizophrenia'. While some *Sd 1* conditions, such as schizoid psychopathy according to the earlier investigators, almost certainly belong to *Sd 3*, other schizophrenic-like conditions may not necessarily distinguish schizophrenics' relatives from either other psychiatric or normal controls. Over-inclusive thinking is one example (McConaghy and Clancy, 1968); and it is unlikely that being *un*married (which some might conceivably call a schizophrenic-like condition) would be found in many studies to be a statistically significant *Sd 3* trait. Some overlap between *Sd 3* and *Sd 1* is illustrated by the overlapping circles of Figure 1b in which *Sd 1* persons are represented by the vertically-hatched circle. The vertically-hatched area within the *Sd 3* circle brings out the point that only some *Sd 3* conditions resemble schizophrenia clinically.

We shall now add another circle to represent psychiatrically abnormal persons (other than schizophrenics) found among the relatives of schizophrenics, that is, what we are calling *Sd 2*. Some of these persons will suffer from *Sd 1* or *Sd 3* disorders, but others will have conditions such as anxiety states which neither resemble schizophrenia clinically nor are generally found significantly more often than in a control group. They are shown by the horizontally-hatched circle in Figure 1(c), which also shows that there may be many *Sd 1* and *Sd 3* individuals who are not closely related to a schizophrenic.

It has been suggested that people classed as schizoid according to each of these definitions might provide a better phenotype for genetic analysis than schizophrenic psychosis, and might give an indication of what is inherited. However, with each the question arises as to how homogeneous the group is genetically. Are all criminals (*Sd 3*), or all over-inclusive thinkers (*Sd 1*), or all anxiety neurotics related to a schizophrenic (*Sd 2*), predicted to be high-risk candidates for developing and transmitting schizophrenia; and if not, what proportion of them are hypothesized as *Sd 4,* that is, schizoid in the genetic sense? Opinions on these points differ and are not well formulated. The search with which we and others are concerned is for an identifiable characteristic, whether dimensional or categorical in form, which is the best attainable indicator of *Sd 4* in a defined population. While one would probably look for such a characteristic within *Sd 1, 2* or *3*, we may note that all schizophrenia genotypes do not reveal themselves easily; very few schizophrenics have a close schizophrenic relative, and a majority are not schizoid premorbidly in either the *Sd 1* or the *Sd 3* sense.

It is obvious that one must exercise considerable caution before claiming to have identified a phenotype which can be substituted for schizophrenia in population genetic studies. However, persons who are schizoid in any of these senses may provide promising leads towards a better understanding of the development of schizophrenia at a biological or any other level. In particular, the relatives of schizophrenics remain a strategic population.

Normality and Schizoidia in Twins of Schizophrenics

Many kinds of data from different kinds of studies on the biological and adoptive relatives of schizophrenics could be used to illustrate the problems so far mentioned. In this paper we shall limit ourselves to the use of some recent twin studies including new analyses of our own Maudsley–Bethlem twins. In another paper (Shields, Heston and Gottesman, 1975) we shall examine the utility of *Sd 1, 2,*

3 and *4* in family and adoptee studies. With co-twins we can note what disorders were found (*Sd 2*), ask which ones were schizophrenic-like (*Sd 1*), and which ones occur more frequently than in control groups (*Sd 3*). Assuming that some of the disorders indicate a schizophrenic genotype, what we call *Sd 4*, do they fit some monogenic or polygenic hypothesis?

The newcomer to this field might believe that the co-twins of identical twins who are schizophrenic should provide *direct* information about what constitutes the range of *Sd 4* phenotypes indicating the presence of a schizophrenic genotype. Even if we ignored the relatively rare non-genetic symptomatic schizophrenias (cf Davison and Bagley, 1969), such a belief would be naive. It does not provide for the role of the environment at any point after fertilization in turning genes on or off differentially in the two members of our human clones, thus rendering their 'effective genotype' non-identical. Reasons for many trait discordances observed in MZ pairs are manifold (cf Gottesman and Shields, 1972; Shields, 1962) and cannot be detailed here. (Although random inactivation of the X chromosomes in female pairs and possibly of some parts of autosomes in all pairs may require some modification of the classical twin method, we will for now assume that all MZ co-twins of true schizophrenics will have a schizophrenic genotype coded in their nuclei and are *Sd 4*.)

In the face of these complications we can understand, on the one hand, Inouye's (1970) conclusion 'that where a monozygotic twin was affected with classical schizophrenia its co-twin was usually distinctly deviated in personality. This agrees well with the early finding by Professor Essen-Möller, and accords with the well-known fact that there exists a peculiar personality deviation among family members of the patients affected with classical schizophrenia (p 95)'. And, on the other hand, Mosher, Stabenau and Pollin's (1973) conclusion that 'Our data from "normal" and non-schizophrenic MZ co-twins of schizophrenics do not support the hypothesis relating Schizoidia to Schizophrenia as we find a similar proportion of schizoid individuals in both groups (p 1175)'. Problems of sample size and follow-up (see especially Belmaker *et al*, 1974) aside, it is no wonder that in a landmark effort to restore descriptive psychiatry to its former credibility and to 'scientize' it Wing, Cooper and Sartorius (1974) found no room for the term schizoid in their final list of 140 key symptoms to describe the 'present state' from a psychiatric interview (they do have social withdrawal as one of their 140 but it feeds into a diagnosis of neurosis; schizoid personality *is* separately listed in their 'Aetiology Schedule' as a kind of personality before first onset).

In some studies the co-twins are as often neurotic as schizophrenic (narrowly diagnosed), and it is then sometimes implied (Kringlen, 1967) that it is therefore only a tendency to mental disorder in general that is inherited. Do we then regard all neurotics as belonging to the schizophrenic spectrum? Clearly not. On the same argument, normality would be part of the spectrum too. In one study (Fischer, 1973) 43 per cent of MZ co-twins were clinically normal, a higher percentage than in any of the three other main categories employed.

Table 1 shows the extent to which normality and non-schizophrenic disorders were diagnosed in seven twin studies. Normality could be paired with severe as well as mild schizophrenia. Differences in the reported 'normality' rates shown may depend partly on the extent of the investigation and standards adopted for what is within the normal range, but they probably also depend considerably on the varying use made by different authors of the ambiguous term schizoid and whether persons with a few schizoid traits were regarded as normal or not. In his original report Tienari (1963) described none of his 16 MZ co-twins as schizophrenic. Six had other psychiatric diagnoses and ten were normal; twelve twins, many of them healthy, displayed schizoid traits. Essen-Möller's (1941) and Inouye's (1970) results are also difficult to tabulate. Both regarded all non-schizophrenic MZ co-twins as schizoid (Inouye) or

TABLE I

Pairwise MZ rates for schizophrenia, schizoid and other psychiatric conditions, and normality in some schizophrenic twin studies

(After Gottesman and Shields, 1972)

Study	Numbers of pairs	% Schizophrenia and ?schizophrenia	% Sd 1 schizoid[a]	% Sd 2 Other disorders[b]	% normal
Luxenburger[c] (1936)	14	72	14	—	14
Rosanoff et al (1934)	41	61	—	7	32
Kallmann (1946)	174	69	21	5	5
Slater (53)	37	64	—	14	22
Kringlen (1967)	45	38	—	29	33
Fischer (1973)	21	48	5	5	43
Gottesman and Shields (1972)	22	50	9	18	23

[a] So diagnosed by investigators.

[b] Includes as examples: alcoholic, psychopath (Kallmann); psychopathic, suicide (Slater); alcoholic, character neurosis (Kringlen).

[c] Only includes co-twins of certain schizophrenics.

as having a characterological trait genetically related to schizophrenia (Essen-Möller). Mosher *et al* (1973) reported that only six
out of fifteen non-schizophrenic MZ co-twins were schizoid, either
in the DSM II sense or in being rated highly in respect of the traits
which Slater (1953) thought were distinctive in the abnormal
relatives in schizophrenics' families. Employing a more liberal interpretation of schizophrenic-like, we considered from the data
presented by Mosher *et al* that at most ten out of sixteen of their co-
twins could be so described. However, Mosher's twin sample was
selected in a nationwide survey for MZ pairs where one member of
the pair was an undoubted schizophrenic and the other was an
undoubted non-schizophrenic and with both parents alive and very
co-operative. The selective biases thus introduced are hard to
evaluate but one result must certainly have been that the co-twins
were an unusually healthy group, as in fact they are compared to the
systematically ascertained twins (but cf Belmaker *et al,* 1974).

Nevertheless, it cannot reliably be claimed, even when using very
liberal criteria, either that nearly 100 per cent of MZ co-twins are
disordered (*Std 2*) or that 100 per cent are schizophrenic or schizoid
personalities (*Sd 1*).

The Maudsley Schizophrenic Twin Series
It may be of interest to examine at first hand the Maudsley Hospital
twin study from Slater's former MRC Psychiatric Genetics Unit
(Gottesman and Shields, 1972) with regard to possible pointers to a
schizophrenic genotype (*Sd 4*) in the co-twins. We shall ask how
many MZ and DZ co-twins of schizophrenics could be conserva-
tively or liberally termed *Sd 1* or *Sd 2;* and we shall discuss the findings in terms of 'schizoid disease' and polygenic theories. The results
are shown in Table 2. A large proportion of the twins were interviewed at follow-up and tested with the Minnesota Multiphasic
Personality Inventory (MMPI).

Of 22 MZ pairs in which a proband was definitely or probably
schizophrenic according to the consensus of six[*] diagnosticians
operating blindfolded with case histories, 11 (50 per cent) were
concordant for schizophrenia, using the same criteria for the co-
twin. As shown below, six co-twins had non-schizophrenic but
psychiatric consensus diagnosis. This gives an *Sd 2* rate of 77 per
cent, using a conventional standard for 'disorder'. However, only
two of these six co-twins had disorders resembling schizophrenia (*Sd
1*) or of a kind that would fall into the 'schizophrenia spectrum' of
Kety *et al* (1968).

---

[*] Eliot Slater, Paul E. Meehl, K. Abe, J. L. T Birley, L. R. Mosher, J. S. Price.

TABLE II

*Disordered (Sd2) and possibly schizoid (Sd1) co-twins of schizophrenics in the
Maudsley Hospital study*

Classification of co-twins	MZ pairs	DZ pairs
a. Schizophrenia or ?schizophrenia (consensus diagnosis)	11	3
b. Other diagnosis: schizoid (clinical	2	1
c. Other diagnosis ?schizoid (MMPI)	—	3
d. Other diagnosis: no evidence of schizoidia	4	5
e. Normal: ?*Sd 4* schizoid (Essen-Möller)	3	—
f. Normal: (?schizoid (MMPI and/or clinical)	—	3
g. Normal: no evidence of schizoidia	2	18
Total		
Sd 2, consensus a+b+c+d	17 (77%)	12 (36%)
Sd 1, maximum a+b+c+e+f	16 (72%)	10 (30%)
Sd 1, (maximum) or Sd 2 a+b+c+d+e+f	20 (91%)	15 (45%)

Probably Sd 1 schizoid disorder. MZ 14B, male, aged 20. Consensus diagnosis was personality disorder (inadequate, hypochondriacal). Some individual judges' diagnoses were (Meehl) pseudoneurotic schizophrenia, (Slater) inadequate personality, and (Essen-Möller) 'Schizophrenia-related personality'. Psychotic appearing MMPI profile (8*56', etc). He had quite fixed ideas about having ulcer disease for which he treated himself, but it had never been found after repeated examinations. His verbatim language from a tape-recorded interview was scored for schizophrenicity using the methods of Gottschalk and Gleser (1969) by Arnold (1971); his G–G score was 5.58. The median score for all schizophrenics in our scored sample of twins was 6.5, for other psychiatric diagnoses, 3.0, and for normals, 1.4; only schizophrenics scored above 6.8.

MZ 16B, male, aged 44. Consensus diagnosis was personality disorder (paranoid). Called a schizotype (Meehl) and schizo-phrenia-related personality (Essen-Möller). He refused both the MMPI and to have the interview tape-recorded; was suspicious, resentful, humourless, irritable, showed little capacity for warmth but was married with one child and had never sought psychological help.

Probably not Sd 1 schizoid disorder. MZ 5B, female, aged 42. Consensus diagnosis was neurotic depression, anxiety. Schizoidia never suspected but her G–G score was 6.03 and her confession of lesbian interests was difficult to integrate with the rest of her personality. MMPI clearly neurotic (31″ 742′ etc).

MZ 9B, female, aged 47. Consensus diagnosis was neurotic depression, anxiety. Schizoidia never suspected clinically, MMPI within normal limits. Her proband sister in our unblindfolded opinion had a symptomatic schizophreniform psychosis caused by a long history of alcoholism.

MZ 18B, female, aged 37. Consensus diagnosis was personality disorder (hysterical), anxiety. Hospitalized 51 weeks for neurosis at age 20, and chronic attender at psychiatric outpatients since. Called pseudoneurotic schizophrenia (Meehl), inadequate personality (Slater), neither normal nor schizoid (Essen-Möller). Refused MMPI but her G–G score was 6.02. Two brothers were psychiatrically hospitalized but our information was inadequate to arrive at diagnoses. Her proband sister had a recurrent schizo-affective illness that responded to reserpine.

MZ 24B, female, aged 40. Consensus diagnosis was post-partum depression. Hospitalized briefly at 31. Very normal at interview as was her MMPI. G–G score was zero.

The brief summaries above may underestimate the prevalence of *Sd 1*. In addition to the two co-twins with probably schizoid disorders, there were three psychiatrically normal co-twins who had schizophrenia-related personalities (*Sd 4*) according to Essen-Möller's review of their histories. That could bring the total with schizoidia, more broadly defined, up to five. The eleven consensus schizophrenic plus the five possibly schizoid co-twins account for 72 per cent of the 22 MZ pairs. In addition there was one co-twin (MZ 4B) of a mild schizophrenic who, at age 39, had an MMPI (98' etc) that would have led to a suspicion of a schizo-affective disorder had she not appeared unremarkable clinically; later—however, her G–G score turned out to be 6.80, the only non-schizophrenic to score that high. The other normal MZ co-twin (MZ 20B) shows nothing of schizoidia at age 46, with a G–G score of 0.93 and a very normal MMPI. Her proband sister has, in our opinion, a symptomatic schizophreniform psychosis associated with thyroid disease; her G–G score was only 1.43 and her MMPI (4' etc) did not even suggest *Sd 1* schizoidia.

In the Maudsley study the premorbid personality of the first (schizophrenic) twin was, so far as we could judge, schizoid or probably so in only 8 of 22 pairs. It is well known that many schizophrenias develop in personalities that are not *Sd 1* schizoid (Bleuler, 1972); we should not expect all MZ co-twins of schizophrenics to be schizoid in the sense of *Sd 1*.

Of the DZ pairs, three out of 33 (9 per cent) were concordant for schizophrenia. Nine co-twins (three of them hospitalized) had other disorders; these were mostly anxiety or depression, sometimes mild and transient. They bring the Sd 2 rate to 36 per cent. Some of these other disorders, it was thought, could be accounted for by environmental stress or by depressive or other non-schizoid personality traits shared with the proband. Only one was generally regarded as a schizoid personality (DSM II sense), but three others among the nine appeared to have a noteworthy schizoid element when the MMPI was considered. Among the normal co-twins a further three might be regarded as schizoid on MMPI and/or other evidence. The maximum concordance for schizophrenia or schizophrenic-like personality (*Sd 1*) is therefore 10/33 (30 per cent) in DZ pairs.

The MZ and DZ concordance rates for *Sd 2*, 77 per cent and 36 per cent respectively, and those for *Sd 1*, 72 per cent and 30 per cent, fall short of the 100 per cent and 50 per cent required according to the dominant 'schizoid disease' (Heston, 1970) hypothesis, which makes an effort to avoid the introduction of 'incomplete expression' that is part of Slater's theory. However, if we count co-twins who either are 'disordered' or are normal but with a possibly schizoid personality, maximum rates of 20/22 (91 per cent) MZ and 15/33 (45 per cent) DZ are achieved, which fall very little short of those predicted. The critic may say, however, that the prediction of 50 per cent affected DZ co-twins makes no allowance for the frequency of a gene supposed to be associated with the abnormalities that gave rise to the maximum rates. For example, if the posited schizoid gene had a frequency in the population of 10 per cent, the expected risk in siblings (including DZ co-twins) of schizophrenics would be 56 per cent rather than the 50 per cent expected with rarer dominant gene conditions. The maximum rates of 91 per cent in MZ and 45 per cent in DZ pairs reported in Table 2 should also allow for the possibilities of environmental phenocopies and of genocopies causing some of the wide range of traits counted as 'affected'. In other words, allowance should be made for false positives contributing to the nice fit with dominant gene theory.

The alternative polygenic model—even less disprovable, according to its critics—looks for a well defined measure which gives good discrimination between MZ and DZ concordance rates (*Sd 3*, MZ v DZ), or which gives consistent estimates of heritability (not necessarily 100 per cent!) (Smith, 1974) independently derived from different kinds of relatives. In the context of the Maudsley study best agreement with the model was achieved with the diagnosis of schizophrenic psychosis itself, using standards that would be regarded as narrow in the US and broad in the UK. Shields and Gottesman (1972) have argued that similar diagnostic standards also work well in other recent twin studies. The search now should be for important contributory aetiological factors; on the genetic side there may be no *single Sd 4* indicator.

Hopes for an Endophenotype

Despite the different diagnostic and strategic procedures and the contradictory findings and interpretations to which we have drawn attention in our discussion of twin studies, perhaps the most promising pointers towards *Sd 4* remain in the area in Figure 1 where our *Sd 1, 2* and *3* circles overlap: it is the broadly schizophrenia-like disorders, such as schizoid character and borderline schizophrenia, which most consistently distinguish the relatives of process schizophrenics from appropriate controls. Beyond that little can be said. After stretching our resources to their utmost extent, we are no nearer to identifying other possible high risk genotypes in schizophrenics' families. In the absence of good objective criteria for schizoid character and other 'borderline' conditions and the consequent lack of adequate epidemiological and family studies of such conditions, it cannot be claimed that we have an improved phenotype for population genetic studies.

At this point it might be helpful to see what can be learned from genetic diseases that are more completely known than schizophrenia. First, diabetes, which in its population genetics is remarkably like schizophrenia. As in schizophrenia, 45–50 per cent of the MZ co-twins of affected persons are concordant. Then, if diabetes is defined as an abnormality in a glucose tolerance test (sometimes performed after an evocative stimulus), some of the remaining co-twins will be 'chemically' diabetic (Gottlieb and Root, 1968). Finally, if the plasma insulin response of co-twins who still seem normal is measured, it appears that nearly 100 per cent will have a measurable abnormality (Cerasi and Luft, 1967; Pyke *et al* 1970). One problem here is that of genetic *expression*. What level of expression will we define as disease? What trait—overt diabetes, an abnormal glucose tolerance curve, or the plasma insulin response—is the best one for genetic analysis? Because severity of disease generally turns out to be important in medical genetics, perhaps all three traits will be useful depending on one's purposes. And even plasma insulin levels are removed from gene action so there will no doubt be other levels of trait definition to come. Although we think that the analogy to diabetes gives much to ponder that we will not make explicit, we will make the main points that expression of a genotype can vary widely indeed and that the comparatively extremely crude level at which the phenotype is assessed in schizophrenia is reason for humility and flexibility, not dogmatism.

A second useful example is the Lesch–Nyhan syndrome. This bizarre X-linked syndrome features a severe neuromuscular disorder, self-mutilation, and mental retardation. The defective enzyme (hypoxanthine guanine phosphoribosyltransferase) has about 0.005 per cent of normal activity in the erythrocytes of affected persons. Now the activity of the same enzyme is deficient in an extraordinary range of other disorders found in Lesch–Nyhan families as well as families located through probands with one or another of those other disorders. Enzyme activity in the range of 0.01 per cent to 0.5 per cent of normal is associated with neurological disorders ranging from retardation to spino-cerebellar syndromes of variable severity. Levels of about 1 per cent of normal are associated with gout (Kelly and Wyngaarden, 1972; Seegmiller, 1972). Certainly some of this clinical and biochemical variability will be associated with different mutations causing different amino acid substitutions in the same enzyme. Some variability can be attributed to differential modification of the enzymes' activity by environmental factors and by the balance of the genome. That the amount of protein translated from a mutant locus varies between families implicating modifying factors of the sort needed has been demonstrated in the case of sickle-cell haemoglobin (Nance and Grove, 1972). The main point is a simple one. There would be no possible way on clinical grounds to group all of the clinical disorders associated with deficiencies in the activity of this one enzyme into one clinical syndrome, not even those disorders appearing in one family. Again, tentativeness and humility are prescribed, but there is the further point that familial clustering of disease provides a logical classification, even if the diseases are very dissimilar at the phenotypic level.

From what we have said about semantics, sampling, and other problems, we may not expect ready agreement about the most valid indicators of the schizoid state genetically (*Sd 4*). We should certainly strive for some better indication of 'what is inherited' than a mid-Atlantic diagnosis of classical schizophrenia. But without further advances in the basic biological sciences, the testing of promising leads will be a laborious and, some might think, a fruitless proceeding. It involves the lengthy follow-up of strategic populations relevant to the transmission of schizophrenia. We have mentioned the desirability of prospective investigation of loosely schizophrenic-like (*Sd 1*) and *Sd 4*-suspect subjects (e.g. the thought-disordered or eccentric or physiologically over-reactive), to discover how many of them and their relatives develop definite schizophrenic psychoses; and we need to know what becomes of the offspring of the matings of couples both of whom suffer from suspected schizophrenia spectrum disorders, both in known 'schizophrenic' families and in unselected samples from the general population.

Because such studies would expend prodigious labour in seeking uncertain rewards, we think the best hope for the resolution of the schizophrenia problem may have to await the finding of a protein which differentiates schizophrenics from others. Short of that, close genetic linkage to a marker gene might be a possibility, despite the acknowledged difficulties (Jayakar, 1970). However, the difficulty in distinguishing 'affected' from 'unaffected' family members, particularly in the younger age groups, would be likely to upset the arithmetic of linkage calculations (too many *Sd 4s* who are not even *Sd 1 or Sd 2*) the attempt might also founder because on a polygenic model there would be too many genes and on a monogenic model too many extraneous influences on expression.

Our hopes lie more with an endophenotype associated with the pathogenesis of schizophrenia. The characteristics of a good biological indicator of this kind have been outlined by Shields and Gottesman (1973). A biological advance may give us a better chance of solving some of the genetic problems in schizophrenia and the schizoid than distilling and juggling clinical categories and test scores. A reliable biochemical measure might help to decide between competing genetic models, discover what psychopathology should be described as schizoid, and identify individuals at high risk of developing a malignant psychosis. In principle, a better understanding of genetic aetiology should lead to improved and rational environmental methods of treatment and prevention.

References

American Psychiatric Association (1968) *Diagnostic and Statistical Manual of Mental Disorders,* (2nd edn). Washington Committee on Nomenclature and Statistics of the American Psychiatric Association.

Arnold, K. (1971) Language in schizophrenics and their twins. Unpub. Ph.D. thesis. University of Minnesota.

Belmaker, R., Pollin, W., Wyatt, R. J. & Cohen, S. (1974) A follow-up of monozygotic twins discordant for schizophrenia. *Arch. Gen Psychiat., 30,* 219–22.

Bleuler, E. (1950) *Dementia Praecox or the Group of Schizophrenias.* Leipzig: Deuticke (1911). Republished, translated by Joseph Zinkin, New York: International Universities Press.

Bleuler, M. (1972) *Die schizphrenen Geistesstörungen im Lichte langjähriger Kranken- und Familiengeschichten.* Stuttgart: Thieme.

Cerasi, E. & Luft, R. (1967) Insulin response to glucose infusion in diabetic and non-diabetic monozygotic twin pairs. Genetic control of insulin response? *Acta Endocrinologica, 55,* 330—45.

Davison, K. & Bagley, C. R. (1969) Schizophrenia-like psychoses associated with organic disorders of the central nervous system: a review of the literature. In *Current Problems in Neuropsychiatry,* British Journal of Psychiatry Special Publication No.4. Ashford, Kent: Headley, 113–184.

Essen-Möller, E. (1941) Psychiatrische Untersuchungen an einer Serie von Zwillingen. *Acta Psychiatrica et Neurologica Scandinavica,* Suppl. 23.

Essen-Möller, E. (1946) The concept of schizoidia. *Monatsschrift für Psychiatrie und Neurologie,* **112,** 258–71.

Fischer, M. (1973) Genetic and environmental factors in schizophrenia. *Acta Psychiat. Scand.,* Suppl. 238.

General Register Office, 1968. *A Glossary of Mental Disorders, Studies on Medical and Population Subjects No 22*. London, Her Majesty's Stationery Office, 1968.

Gottesman, I. I. (1974) Developmental genetics and ontogenetic psychology: overdue detente and propositions from a matchmaker. In *Minnesota Symposium on Child Psychology* (ed. A. Pick) Minneapolis: University of Minnesota Press.

Gottesman, I. I. & Shields, J. (1967) A polygenic theory of schizophrenia, *Proceedings of the National Academy of Science*, **58**, 199–205.

Gottesman, I. I. & Shields, J. (1972) *Schizophrenia and Genetics: a Twin Study Vantage Point*. New York: Academic Press.

Gottesman, I. I. Shields, J. & Heston, L. L. (1976) Characteristics of the twins of schizophrenics as fallible indicators of schizoidia. *Acta Geneticae medicae et Gemellologiae*, **25**, 225—36.

Gottlieb, M. S. & Root, H. F. (1968) Diabetes mellitus in twins. *Diabetes*, **17**, 693–704.

Gottschalk, L. A. & Gleser, G. C. (1969) *The Measurement of Psychological States through the Content Analysis of Verbal Behaviour*. Berkeley: University of California Press.

Heston, L. L. (1966) Psychiatric disorders in foster home reared children of schizophrenic mothers. *British Journal of Psychiatry*, **122**, 819–25.

Heston, L. L. (1970) The genetics of schizophrenic and schizoid disease. *Science*, **167**, 249–56.

Inouye, E. (1970) Personality deviation seen in monozygotic co-twins of the index cases with classical schizophrenia. *Acta Psychiat. Scand.*, **219**, 90–6.

Jayakar, S. D. (1970). On the detection and estimation of linkage between a locus influencing a quantitative character and a marker locus. *Biometrics*, **26**, 451–64.

Kahn, E. (1923) Studien uber Vererbung und Entstehung geistiger Störungen. IV. Schizoid und Schizophrenie im Erbgang. *Monographien aus dem Gesamtgebiete der Neurologie und Psychiatrie*, 36.

Kallmann, F. J. (1938) *The Genetics of Schizophrenia*. New York: Augustin.

Kallmann, F. J. (1946) The genetic theory of schizophrenia. *American Journal of Psychiatry*, **103**: 309–22.

Kelley, W. N. & Wyngaarden, J. B. (1972) The Lesch–Nyhan syndrome. In *The Metabolic Basis of Inherited Disease* (3rd ed), (ed S. B. Stanbury, J. B. Wyngaarden & D. S. Fredrickson. New York: McGraw-Hill.

Kety, S. S., Rosenthal, D., Wender, P. H. & Schulsinger F. (1968) The types and prevalence of mental illness in the biological and adoptive families of adopted schizophrenics. In *The Transmission of Schizophrenia* (ed. D. Rosenthal & S. S. Kety. Oxford: Pergamon, 345–62.

Kety, S. S. Rosenthal, D., Wender, P. H., Schulsinger, F. & Jacobsen B. (1975) Mental illness in the biological and adoptive families of adopted individuals who have become schizophrenic: a preliminary report based upon psychiatric interviews. In *Genetic Research in Psychiatry* (ed R. Fieve, D. Rosenthal & H. Brill. Baltimore: Johns Hopkins Press.

Kretschmer, E. (1921) *Körperbau und Charakter*, (1st edn). Berlin: Springer.

Kringlen, E. (1967) *Heredity and Environment in the Functional Psychoses*. London: Heinemann.

Luxenberger, H. (1936) Untersuchungen an schizophrenen Zwillingen und ihren Geschwistern zur Prüfung der Realität von Manifestationsschwankungen. *Zeitschrift für die Gesamte Neurologie und Psychiatrie*, **154**, 351–94.

McConaghy, N & Clancy, M. (1968) Familial relationships of allusive thinking in university students and their parents. *British Journal of Psychiatry*, **114**, 1079–87.

Macfarlane, J. W., Allen, L. & Honzik, M. P. (1962) *Behaviour Problems of Normal Children*. Berkeley: University of California Press.

Meehl, P. E. (1962) Schizotaxia, schizotypy, Schizophrenia. *American Psychologist,* **17,** 827–38.

Meehl, P. E. (1964) Manual for use with checklist of schizotypic signs. Unpublished manuscript, University of Minnesota Medical School, Minneapolis.

Meehl, P. E. (1973) *Psychodiagnosis. Selected Papers,* Minneapolis: Univ of Minn. Press.

Meehl, P. E. & Rosen, A. (1955) Antecedent probability and the efficiency of psychometric signs, patterns, or cutting scores. *Psychological Bulletin,* 52, 194–216.

Michael, C. M., Morris, D. P. & Soroker, E. (1957) Follow-up studies of shy, withdrawn children. II: Relative incidence of schizophrenia. *American Journal of Orthopsychiatry,* **27,** 331–7.

Morris, D. P., Soroker, E. & Burruss, G. (1954) Follow-up studies of shy, withdrawn children. I: Evaluation of later adjustment. *American Journal of Orthopsychiatry,* **24,** 743–54.

Mosher, L. R., Stabenau, J. R. & Pollin, W. (1973) Schizoidness in the non-schizophrenic identical co-twins of schizophrenics. *Excerpta Med. Int. Cong,* Series 274, 1164–76.

Nance, W. E., & Grove, J. (1972) Genetic determination of phenotypic variation in sickle cell trait. *Science,* **177,** 716–17.

Ødegaard, Ø. (1946) Marriage and mental disease. *J. ment. Sci,* 92, 35–9.

Planansky, K. (1972) Phenotypic boundaries and genetic specificity in schizophrenia. In *Genetic Factors in 'Schizophrenia'* (Ed A. R. Kaplan), Springfield, Ill.: Thomas, 141–72.

Pyke, D. A., Cassar, J., Todd, J. & Taylor, K. W. (1970) Glucose tolerance and serum insulin in identical twins of diabetics. *British Medical Journal,* iv, 649–51.

Rado, S. (1962) Theory and therapy: the theory of schizotypal organization and its application to the treatment of decompensated schizotypal behaviour. In *Psychoanalysis of Behaviour,* Vol. II (ed S. Rado). New York: Grune & Stratton, 127–40.

Rosenthal, D. (1975) Evidence for a spectrum of schizophrenic disorders. Unpublished manuscript.

Rosanoff, A. J., Handy, L. M., Plesset, I. R. and Brush, S. (1934) The etiology of so called schizophrenic psychoses with special reference to their occurrence in twins. *American Journal of Psychiatry,* **91,** 725–62.

Seegmiller, J. E. (1972) Lesch–Nyhan syndrome and the X-linked uric acidurias. *Hospital Practice,* **April 1972,** 79–90.

Shields, J. (1962) *Monozygotic Twins Brought Up Apart and Brought Up Together.* Oxford University Press.

Shields, J. (1971) Concepts of heredity for schizophrenia. In *The Origin of Schizophrenia* (ed M. Bleuler & J. Angst, Bern: Huber, 59–75.

Shields, J. & Gottesman, I. I. (1972) Cross-national diagnosis of schizophrenia in twins. *Archives of General Psychiatry,* **27,** 725–30.

Shields, J. & Gottesman, I. I. (1973) Genetic studies of schizophrenia as signposts to biochemistry. In *Biochemistry and Mental Illness* (ed L. L. Iversen & S. Rose). London: Biochemical Society, 165—174.

Shields, J. Heston, L. L. & Gottesman, I. I. (1975) Schizophrenia and the schizoid: the problem for genetic analysis. In R. Fieve, D. Rosenthal & H. Brill. *Genetic Research in Psychiatry,* Baltimore: Johns Hopkins Press, 167–97.

Slater, E. (with the assistance of J. Shields) (1953) Psychotic and neurotic illnesses in twins. *Medical Research Council Special Report Series No. 278,* London: Her Majesty's Stationery Office.

Slater, E. (1958) The monogenic theory of schizophrenia. *Acta Genetica et Statistica Medica,* **8,** 50–6.

Slater, E. & Cowie, V. A. (1971) *The Genetics of Mental Disorders.* London: Oxford University Press.

Smith, C. (1974) Concordance in twins: methods and interpretation. *Amer J. Hum Genet.*, **26**, 454–66.

Stevens, B. C. (1969) *Marriage and Fertility of Women Suffering from Schizophrenia or Affective Disorders.* London: Oxford University Press.

Tieenari, P. (1963) Psychiatric illnesses in identical twins. *Acta Psychiatrica Scandinavica,* Suppl. 171.

Wing, J. K., Cooper, J. E. & Sartorius, N. (1974) *The Measurement and Classification of Psychiatric Symptoms.* London: Cambridge University Press.

Zerbin-Rüdin, E. (1967) Endogene Psychosen. In *Humangenetik, ein kurzes Handbuch,* Vol. V/2 (ed P. E. Becker). Stuttgart: Thieme, 446–577.

GENETIC FACTORS IN
BEHAVIOURAL DISORDERS

David Rosenthal

Introduction

My admired friend and colleague, Eliot Slater, has long been concerned with mental disorders and their origins, and the quality of life for the sick or well, for the living or the dying. Because of his great concern for science and humanitarianism, which has had an impact on me and many others, I offer herein a paper which in a small way reflects some of his lifelong concerns, and in which I 'come down strong on one side of the fence or the other', a remark he applied to himself repeatedly.

Many among us may not have thought of mental illness as one of the major factors contributing to current public agitation, yet it does provide a deeply unsettling input into national frustrations, whether in regard to fiscal matters, manpower, the quality of work and of life itself or the tolerance or intolerance of deviant behaviours that eventually shapes and provides direction to changes in our moral and legal codes, including matters of sex, violence, familial and social class relationships, and even relations between the races.

Let me give you some idea of the magnitude of the mental illness problem. First of all, the term mental illness includes a wide range of diagnostic syndromes. These include schizophrenia, manic-depressive psychoses and other affective disorders, psychoneuroses of various kinds, psychosomatic disorders in which psychological problems play an important role, sexual disabilities and deviations accompanied by psychological distress, psychopathic personalities—especially those accompanied by crime and delinquency; alcoholism, drug addiction, suicide; mental disturbances in children—including early infantile autism, childhood schizophrenia, the hyperkinetic syndrome often referred to as minimal brain dysfunction, symptomatic disturbances such as reading disability, and speech defects that have emotional accompaniments, especially stuttering; some syndromes involving loss of sphincter control; mental deficiencies of all kinds; mental disorders associated with brain aberrations, as in epilepsy, brain trauma, and senility; or disorders associated with normal life processes involving metabolic change—as in postpartum and menopausal psychoses.

According to a National Institute of Mental Health report based on the year 1967, approximately half a million hospital beds in the USA were occupied by mental patients. One half of these, or a quarter of a million beds, were occupied by patients with the most severe mental illness, schizophrenia. However, these were prevalence figures. Most studies indicate that the actual incidence of schizophrenia in the population is approximately 1 per cent. Therefore, in a population of 200 million people, we have approximately 2 million schizophrenics. Since there are at most only a quarter of a million schizophrenics in the hospital at any single time (the figure is lower now), there are more than one and three-quarter million schizophrenic or potentially schizophrenic hospitalizable patients currently walking the street in their own inimitable way. The cost of schizophrenia to the country is said to be 14,000 million dollars a year. But that is only part of the picture. For every hospitalizable schizophrenic, there are many more people in the community who have a schizophrenic-like type of disorder which is not severe enough to require hospitalization. These individuals are called borderline or pseudoneurotic schizophrenic, schizoid, paranoid, or simply cold, distant and inadequate, or odd and eccentric.

Concerning depression, 90,000 people with this disorder were hospitalized in 1967 and many times more never found their way to the hospital. With respect to suicide, at least once every minute someone in the United States tried to kill himself, and once every 24 minutes the attempt was successful.

According to the latest counts, there are 9 million people in the United States with a serious drinking problem, or about one in every 22 persons, whose annual costs to the nation include 10,000 million dollars, half of all arrests, and 25,000 highway deaths. An estimated 200,000 new cases develop each year.

Concerning crime and delinquency, on any given day there were half a million persons in jails and prisons in 1967, and prison crowding has got worse. It was estimated that approximately one child in five between the ages of ten and seventeen would one day appear before a juvenile court judge. Homicide was the fifteenth leading cause of death in the nation, and the cost of crime to the country was said to be in excess of 20,000 million dollars each year. First admission rates and resident population rates in mental hospitals for children under the age of fifteen were increasing alarmingly.

Concerning institutionalization for mental retardation, there were 13,000 first admissions of children in the year 1967, and 78,000 children were residents in such institutions at the end of the year. In addition, about one child in every twenty is now thought to have minimal brain dysfunction.

Psychoneurosis is so prevalent in the population that it is almost impossible to estimate. In a study of school-age twins carried out in London (Shields, 1954), more than half (54 per cent) were diagnosed as psychoneurotic and only 18 per cent had 'no neurotic traits of significance'. In a study of a population of 110,000 adults in midtown Manhattan (Srole et al, 1962), it was again found that only about 18 per cent of the entire sample were classified as 'well' or essentially symptom-free, and almost a quarter (23.4 per cent) or about 25,740 in this one small section of the borough were found to be 'seriously impaired'. Thus, few families in the nation are entirely free of mental disorders. Indeed, it may very well be that the so-called 'normal' person, with respect to mental health, does not represent a norm at all, but rather an ideal—relatively rare—that most of us would like to achieve.

One reason for presenting the above information regarding the high population frequencies of the various behavioural disorders is to assure the reader that we are dealing with common disorders, in which the problems of genetic analysis differ from those diseases which involve genes of high specificity. On this issue, I can do no better than quote from an article entitled 'The genetic basis of common disease' by Edwards (1963).

> Except for the more common haemoglobinopathies and some variants occasionally revealed by treatment with drugs, genes of high specificity have not been shown to be either necessary or sufficient to cause the development of any common disease. Plausible attempts have been made, with or without Procrustean algebra, to relate the development of many common diseases including diabetes, hypertension and schizophrenia to specific genes. The apparent success of these attempts in no way implies that alternative explanations are less appropriate. Conventional statistical analyses are of little value in discriminating between discontinuous variation related to abrupt difference of genotype relevant to one locus and quasi-continuous variation related to underlying continuous variation due to the unresolved effects of numerous genes, environment or their even more complex interactions.

Thus, Edwards puts us on notice that, in evaluating the genetics of the behavioural disorders, we have no reason to be confident that they will involve genes of high specificity, or that a single-gene theory will be more or less applicable to them than a theory involving multiple genes of smaller effect. We can say at the outset that

Edwards' generalization holds true for all the behavioural disorders in the sense that no specific genetic theory in regard to any of them has been clearly established. Since Edwards assures us that we are not likely to resolve such differences of opinion, and since all the evidence that we have to date seems to bear him out, we will now concern ourselves primarily with the issue of how we can tell in the behavioural disorders whether genes play any specific role at all.

We must first note the nature of the phenotypes with which we are dealing. They are all defined by behaviours that are not always present, that shade off into one another, sometimes almost imperceptibly, that are often difficult to define precisely, and that vary from time to time and person to person both in the manner and the degree of their expression. Thus, it is not surprising that agreement on whether the disorder is present in a given subject is less than perfect. In fact, the reliability of phenotype determination is much lower than that found in most other common diseases. Investigators in the field must tolerate an appreciable margin of diagnostic error, which in turn varies from study to study.

In the more distant past, genetic analysis of the behavioural disorders has been predicated on the following (sometimes tacit) assumptions:

(1) If the frequency of the disorder is greater in the relatives of an index case as compared to the frequency in a control group or in the population at large, the disorder is inherited. This assumption fails to address itself to the possibility that rearing and behavioural patterns within the family could lead to the increased incidence in the relatives of index cases.

(2) If the concordance rate for the disorder is higher in monozygotic (MZ) than in dizygotic (DZ) twins, the disorder is inherited. With respect to twins, there is rarely any reason to expect DZ twins to have *higher* concordance rates than MZ twins, even on environmentalist grounds. Also, the assumption made in regard to twins is that intra-pair differences in environmental factors are the same for both MZ and DZ twins. However, many investigators have shown that the psychological aspects of being an identical twin are quite different from those involving DZ twinship. Thus, in both family and twin studies, the possible genetic and environmental factors are confounded, and one can draw conclusions about them only at considerable risk. To be on more secure ground, it is helpful to separate the genetic and the rearing or other implicated psychological variables that might be confounded in the families or in the twinships. This is best done by examining individuals related to a proband but separated from that proband early in life through formal adoption. With these points in mind, I will try to review

briefly the most salient information we have on the major behavioural disorders.

Schizophrenia*

With a few rare exceptions, the incidence of schizophrenia in the first degree relatives of schizophrenic probands is appreciably higher than the incidence of the disorder in control groups or in the population at large. Concordance rates for the disorder are almost always higher in MZ than in DZ twins, and in different studies range from 6 per cent to 86 per cent for MZ twins, with a median value of approximately 50 per cent. It was possible to compile from various sources, some not systematically obtained, MZ twins who have been separated relatively early in life, at least one of whom was schizophrenic. Among them the concordance rate for schizophrenia was actually *higher* than the median rate reported for MZ twins in the systematically sampled studies, probably because of sampling bias. With respect to studies involving adoption, we can now report that all five of the studies done to date find a higher incidence of schizophrenic disorder in the separated biological relatives of schizophrenic probands than in selected comparison groups. Thus, all the major evidence points to the implication of genetic factors in this disorder, and this conclusion now finds common acceptance.

With respect to the mode of genetic transmission, some investigators have advocated a single-gene theory involving dominance or partial dominance, some a theory of recessiveness, and some have advocated two-gene theories with both dominant, both recessive, or one dominant and the other recessive. Others favour a polygenic theory.

Many investigators have considered it likely that schizophrenia, like mental deficiency, will prove to be a composite of different genetic disorders, some of which will be associated with different single genes of high specificity. However, when we examine the distribution of schizophrenia within families with respect to the three major subclassifications of schizophrenia, paranoid, catatonic, and hebephrenic, we find that, although there is a correlation with respect to subtype, in fact all of the subtypes occur at far better than chance frequencies within the same families. Thus, if a theory of heterogeneity proves to be correct, it probably will not involve the subtype distinctions as such, but might instead be based on some other characteristics of this disorder. For example, some Russian investigators (see Vartanyan and Gindilis, 1972) claim to find some sex linkage with different clinical courses in schizophrenia. They

---

*From this point on, except where other references are cited, the data and original sources on which these summaries of findings are based can be found in Rosenthal (1970).

state that when the illness has its onset in youth and takes a chronic, deteriorating course it occurs approximately one and a half to two times more frequently in men than in women. On the other hand, if the illness is periodic and is manifested as temporally discrete, acute attacks, with complete recession of symptoms during remission and with only slight personality changes, the frequency of this disorder is about two to two and a half times more frequent in women than in men. The authors also claimed to find a form of schizophrenia which they call intermittent-progressive, which clinically is intermediate between the chronic and the recurrent forms, and that this form occurs with equal frequency in both sexes. However, American investigators have not been inclined to look at schizophrenia in this way, and the findings of the Soviet investigators clearly require replication.

There is, however, another distinction regarding the schizophrenic disorders which does seem to involve some genetic heterogeniety. For example, one type of acute psychotic reaction has been called *reactive schizophrenia*. In this disorder, the individual has a single attack, of fairly short duration, in which the symptoms of the psychosis clearly have a schizophrenic quality, but the individual recovers spontaneously without showing the signs of defect that are found in chronic schizophrenics. Recent studies indicate that this form of schizophrenic-like reaction is not related genetically to chronic schizophrenia (Kety *et al,* 1968; Rosenthal *et al,* 1971), a fact that had been accepted by European psychiatrists long ago.

Evidence has been accumulating to the effect that various other schizophrenic-like disorders *are* genetically related to chronic schizophrenia. These include borderline or pseudoneurotic schizophrenia, and at least some severe paranoid and schizoid individuals. Such findings suggest that schizophrenia is a graded character and not an all-or-none type of illness. As a matter of fact, one can examine a group of chronic schizophrenics and rank the individuals in it according to severity of the illness with high reliability. However, although we can demonstrate the graded character of schizophrenic disorders, we are not able to affirm this as proof that multiple genes of small effect are responsible for this seemingly continuous distribution. It is possible that a single major gene underlies the disorder, but that various modifiers and environmental factors make for the gradation of severity manifested. At present, there is a ferment of research activity, accompanied by high optimism, aimed at finding a specific metabolic defect in schizophrenia.

A finding of genetic factors in schizophrenia must be seen in conjunction with a long-known fact that schizophrenics have a lower fertility rate than the general population. Investigators have questioned why the genes for schizophrenia have flourished to the extent that one person in a hundred manifests the illness, and why the incidence of schizophrenia in the population has tended to remain constant, as best we can tell, in the face of reduced fitness. Several original speculations have been proposed to explain these findings, but all have failed to evoke a consensus in their favour. Since the introduction of phenothiazine compounds to treat schizophrenia, the fertility of schizophrenics has been increasing, and approaching the fertility of the population at large. This development appals eugenicists, but the matter lies there at the present time.

Homosexuality

The most common form of sexual deviation is homosexuality. In the few studies examining the families of homosexuals, the investigators found an unusually high frequency of psychopathological conditions of many kinds, as well as turbulent interpersonal relations within the families. One clearly gets the picture that the families, and the homosexuals among them, are not at all gay—in the old-fashioned sense of that maligned little word—and neither was there any sense of liberation in these families. As these studies were carried out in different countries from five to thirty years ago, it may be that in the more tolerant society of today we might find much less emotional turmoil in families with homosexuals.

The major evidence for a genetic factor in homosexuality comes from twin studies, in which the median concordance rate for MZ pairs hovers around 50 per cent, as compared with 8 per cent for DZ pairs. Sampling problems have always been especially difficult in studies of homosexuality, for apparent reasons; but even when we make allowances for sampling bias we must still accord appreciable weight to the evidence from twins.

Strangely, perhaps we confront some difficulties when we have to make decisions about whom we should call a homosexual. Should anyone who has ever had a homosexual experience be counted as a positive case? Kinsey et al (1948) reported that 37 per cent of their male subjects had overt homosexual experiences—to the point of orgasm. Four per cent were exclusively homosexual. Eight per cent had been exclusively homosexual during a three-year period; and fully 18 per cent were more homosexual than heterosexual. Even if we again encounter sampling bias in the Kinsey studies, it is nevertheless clear that homosexual behaviour is so common among American males that, with respect to the definition of this graded phenotype, we may well ask with tongue in cheek, where is the cutoff point!

There is an interesting relationship between homosexuality and schizophrenia. In a study of schizophrenics, investigators found that more than seven out of ten schizophrenic males had problems around heterosexuality; 51 per cent manifested overt homosexual concerns while they were actively psychotic, and 24 per cent had had recorded homosexual experiences. In the largest study of homosexual male MZ twins, the investigator found that six of his forty pairs, or 15 per cent, were concordant for schizophrenia, and that many others were diagnosed as schizoid.

Not only do we have this clinical overlap between schizophrenia and homosexuality, but homosexual disturbance, like schizophrenia, leads to markedly reduced fertility. If there is a genetic factor in homosexuality, as the evidence suggests, we ought to have some explanation of why the genes have become so prevalent, and why homosexuality continues to occur at such high rates in the face of markedly impaired fitness.

A recent study has provided us with a possible biological explanation regarding male homosexuality (Kolodny et al, 1971). The investigators found that male homosexuals had plasma testosterone levels significantly below those of heterosexual controls and also had a significantly lower sperm count. As yet, this study has not been replicated; nor is it possible to state with certainty whether the reduced levels found in the homosexual group reflected a possible genetic aetiology or had some other explanation.

Manic-Depressive Disorders and Alcoholism

The second major group of psychoses has traditionally been called manic-depressive insanity. Whereas schizophrenia has primarily been thought of as a cognitive disorder, manic-depressive psychosis is considered to be a disorder of affect, with both its excitatory and depressive conditions combined into a single diagnostic entity. Evidence for a genetic anlage in the affective psychoses comes primarily from family and twin studies. All of the investigations have methodological flaws, but the combined data point strongly enough toward a genetic contribution to these disorders for it to seem unlikely that methodological errors alone could account for the findings. Calculated heritabilities have been quite high, and the possible mode of genetic transmission has been debated vigorously over the years. Most investigators have favoured the hypothesis of a single dominant gene with only moderately reduced penetrance.

In recent years, however, investigators have tended to divide the manic-depressive disorders into three main subtypes. Two are called unipolar; they comprise individuals whose illness has been only depressive or only manic. The third subtype is called bipolar and comprises individuals who have had both manic and depressive episodes. These investigators (Perris, 1966; Angst, 1966; Dunner et al, 1970) report that in relatives of unipolar patients there occurs a high incidence of unipolar illness, but only a low incidence of bi-polar illness. In contrast, relatives of bipolar patients have a higher incidence of bipolar illness than do unipolar patients. The rates reported differ appreciably but the tendency of the findings has been fairly consistent. However, in MZ twins concordant for affective disorders the subtype forms are discordant in one out of every four pairs (Winokur, et al, 1969; Zerbin-Rüdin, 1967).

Manic-depressive disorders, like schizophrenic disorders, tend to represent a broad spectrum of behaviours, from mild depressions that seem to be triggered by environmental events to the flagrant forms of the psychosis which may include delusions or even hallucinations. Although most investigators have thought the incidence of manic-depressive disorders to be slightly less than the incidence of schizophrenia, one investigator estimates that the incidence of affective illness in the American population is more than 2 per cent. Differences in estimates depend again on which disorders are included in the phenotype.

One consistent finding is that women have these disorders more frequently than men, suggesting the possibility of sex linkage. Two investigators (Perris, 1966; Angst, 1966) have noted an excess of affective disorders in the female relatives of unipolar cases, and Perris found more mother–son pairs than father–son pairs for uni-polar forms of the illness but not for bipolar forms, suggesting that the unipolar form involves an X-linked dominant gene. Other investigators (Reich et al, 1969; Winokur et al, 1969) have reported quite different findings, including an excess of affected females in the first degree relatives of bipolar patients, and no father–son pairs at all, but a fairly appreciable number of mother–son pairs. Thus, these studies are contrary to the others. One group of investigators (Winokur et al, 1969) used colour blindness as an X-chromosome marker in two families with bipolar forms of the illness and reported that the affective disorder in the families was consistently associated with the X-chromosome marker. Thus, it appears that we are advancing our knowledge of the genetics of the affective disorders, but the picture is not yet clear. We might add parenthetically that recent advances in the pharmacological treatment of the affective disorders also encourage us to consider the unipolar and bipolar forms of affective disorder as separate diagnostic entities.

Investigators have also found an association between affective disorders and alcoholism. In one study, about one out of every ten fathers of an affective disorder proband was found to be an alcoholic. This finding is of some interest because studies of alcoholism in twins have suggested a genetic component for this disorder as well. Is it possible that there is some genetic overlap between the affective disorders and alcoholism? Or may it be that individuals suffering from affective disorders or their close kin are prone to resort to alcohol to dispel the deep despair experienced by the subjects and their relatives during periods of depression?

Criminality and Psychoneurosis

It has long been suspected that some inherited factor is associated with criminality. Evidence to support such a view has come primarily from twin studies. It would be surprising indeed to find a single major gene underlying the propensity to crime. In fact, a poorly defined trait such as criminality, if it has any genetic component at all, is most likely to be associated with a number of other genetically influenced traits or disorders. In this sense, criminality provides us with the possibility of demonstrating a type of behavioural disorder that clearly involves genetic heterogeneity.

Let me list a number of these.

(1) A number of studies have reported a higher incidence of EEG abnormalities in criminals than in the population at large. Such abnormalities often have a genetic origin. The EEG abnormalities may be associated with poor impulse control and with bad judgement, which lead to crime.

(2) Many criminals have a low IQ. The IQ is well known to have a high heritability. It can be shown that low IQ individuals, placed in an environment where they can be readily influenced by smarter individuals with crime intentions, are easily led into crime.

(3) Criminals tend to be predominately mesomorphic. Individuals with this type of body build, which clearly has a strong inherited component, tend to be strong, tough, aggressive, and relatively fearless. They seem to have a low tolerance of frustration and they are quick to fight for or take what they want; such characteristics readily bring them into conflict with the law.

(4) Many crimes are committed by individuals who are psychotic or near-psychotic. We have already seen that the major and most common psychoses are associated with some genetic factor. Therefore, such genes can contribute as well to criminality.

(5) Chromosomal aneuploidy may also contribute toward a propensity to crime; the XYY individuals who have received considerable publicity in recent years for their violent crimes may have been reflecting the influence of the extra Y chromosome. However, it is important to note that XXY individuals also manifest an increased tendency towards criminality. We certainly do not associate the X chromosome with criminality. Therefore, it is possible that in the latter group the affected individuals are driven to criminality because of the psychological distress accompanying the physical deviations resulting from the additional X chromosome.

(6) Many individuals carry a psychiatric diagnosis of psychopathic personality. It is this group that probably contributes the highest proportion of individuals whose criminality has some underlying genetic component. A recent adoption study of psychopathic personality provides the best evidence that this type of behavioural syndrome is heritable (Schulsinger, 1969). The prevalence rates of this personality syndrome have been reported to be anywhere from one half of one per cent to 15 per cent in different populations.

Thus, we are able to list at least half a dozen ways in which different types of genes can contribute to a common behavioural disorder.

The most common behavioural disorder of all is psychoneurosis, and although many studies report higher concordance for MZ than DZ twins with respect to various neurotic traits, genetic research on the disorder itself has been relatively meagre and the studies of clinical psychoneurosis that are available have not been methodologically strong. It seems likely, however, that psychoneurosis also represents a heterogeneous collection of disorders involving a wide range of genotypes or polygenic systems.

Summary

There is sufficient evidence for genetic factors in all the behavioural disorders for us to take the genetic hypothesis seriously, but some of the various disorders may not be genetically independent of one another, which makes genetic analysis even more complicated than we had reason to expect. Although the task of genetic analysis is difficult, we seem to be making some progress. Any success that we may be able to achieve in such analysis will not only yield a gratifying scientific payoff but may help as well to alleviate some of the most prevalent, costly and socially debilitating problems that confront the human species today.

References

Angst, J. (1966) *Zur Ätiologie und Nosologie endogener depressiver Psychosen.* Monographien aus dem Gesamtgebiete der Neurologie und Psychiatrie, Heft 112. Berlin: Springer-Verlag.

Dunner, D. L., Gershon, E. S. & Goodwin, F. K. (1970) Heritable factors in the severity of affective illness. Presented at the Annual Meeting of the American Psychiatric Association, May.

Edwards, J. H. (1963) The genetic basis of common disease. *Amer. J. Med.,* 34, 627–38.

Kety, S. S., Rosenthal, D., Wender, P. H. & Schulsinger, F. (1968) The types and prevalence of mental illness in the biological and adoptive families of adopted schizophrenics. In *The Transmission of Schizophrenia* (ed. D. Rosenthal and S. S. Kety). London: Pergamon Press, 345–62.

Kinsey, A. C., Pomeroy, W. B. & Martin, C. E. (1948) *Sexual Behaviour in the Human Male*. Philadelphia: W. B. Saunders.

Kolodny, R. C., Masters, W. H., Hendryx, J. & Toro, G. (1971) Plasma testosterone and semen analysis in male homosexuals. *New Eng. J. of Med.*, 285, 1170–4.

National Institute of Mental Health (1967) Report. In *The Advancement of Knowledge for the Nation's Health*. US Dept. HEW, PHS, July, 110–25.

Perris, C. (1966) A study of bipolar (manic-depressive) and unipolar recurrent depressive psychoses. *Acta Psychiat. Scand.*, 42, Suppl. 194.

Reich, T., Clayton, P. J. & Winokur, G. (1969) Family history studies: V. The genetics of mania. *Amer. J. Psychiat.*, 125, 1358–69.

Rosenthal, D. (1970) *Genetic Theory and Abnormal Behaviour*. New York: McGraw-Hill.

Rosenthal, D., Wender, P. H., Kety, S. S., Welner, J. & Schulsinger, F. (1971) The adopted-away offspring of schizophrenics. *Amer. J. Psychiat.*, 128, 307–11.

Schulsinger, F. (1969) Psychopathy: heredity and environment. Unpublished manuscript, Copenhagen, Denmark.

Shields, J. (1954) Personality differences and neurotic traits in normal twin school-children. *Eugenics Rev.*, 45, 213–46.

Srole, L., Langner, T. S., Michael, S. T., Opler, M. K. & Rennie, T. A. C. (1962) *Mental Health in the Metropolis: The Midtown Manhattan Study, Volume 1*. New York: McGraw-Hill.

Vartanyan, M. E. & Gindilis, V. M. (1972) The role of chromosomal aberrations in the clinical polymorphism of schizophrenia. *Int. J. Ment. Health*, 1, 93–106.

Winokur, G., Clayton, P. J. & Reich, T. (1969) *Manic-Depressive Illness*. St Louis: C. V. Mosby Co.

Zerbin-Rüdin, E. (1967) Endogene Psychosen. In *Humangenetik*, P. E. Becker (ed.) Vol. 5, 2nd Section. Stuttgart: Georg Thiem Verlag.

A DIAGNOSTICIAN DIAGNOSED
DIAGNOSTIC PRACTICE IN PSYCHIATRIC GENETICS STUDIES

James Shields†

Since November 1947 I have had the pleasure and privilege of working with Eliot Slater as chief, colleague and friend. When, as a layman, I first read the files on the twins he had investigated before the war I was perplexed by the confusion and disagreement about psychiatric diagnosis—a problem which is still with us all. Take Case 11 as an example (Slater, 1953, p. 122). The proband's hospital diagnosis was recent melancholia; she was depressed and agitated and said she had done more wicked, dirty, filthy things than anybody in the world had ever thought of. Slater's diagnosis was schizophrenia; he noted her disconnected speech, inappropriate affect and odd mannerisms. She said that people could read her mind and that when she listened to the wireless it was all about what she had done. The difference in diagnosis was usually that way round—the hospital diagnosing melancholia and Slater schizophrenia—though Case 162, p. 273, is an exception. The situation was even more confusing with Case 11's identical twin: the medical certificate gave the diagnosis as puerperal mania, the hospital's report to the Board of Control said she suffered from recent melancholia, while Slater's diagnosis made from case notes after her death was schizophrenia.

When I visited the London County Council's mental hospitals to discover what had become of these patients I began to appreciate Slater's skill as a diagnostician. More often than not the hospital diagnosis had now been switched from recent melancholia to schizophrenia; for instance, proband 11, still in hospital, had expressed the belief that Jesus worked in the laundry. Her speech and thought were said to have been disorganized and she was at times hallucinated and sometimes apathetic and indifferent, verging

†James Shields died in 1978.

34

on stupor. It is worth noting that, depending on who made the diagnosis and when, the pair could be diagnostically discordant, or concordant for either schizophrenia or affective psychosis.

Another example is Case 2 (p. 176). The proband's medical certificate and the hospital record in 1935 both gave the diagnosis as melancholia. Eight months later Slater diagnosed schizophrenia. Though there was an unquestionable depressive affect, there was no self-reproach. She was suspicious and wrapped up in herself; there was a stereotyped repetitiveness about her gestures and she was full of abnormal ideas, believing for instance that the doctors could all read her brain and that her brother was still putting poison in her medicine. In 1947 she was still in hospital but the diagnosis had been revised. Her monozygotic twin was normal when seen in 1935 but in 1947 had recently committed suicide, having been depressed since being told she had a growth in her groin.

In commenting on the published case histories, Slater discusses some of the diagnostic and genetic issues. In Case 11 he considers schizophrenia to be much the most likely diagnosis of both the twins, despite the affective features early on. Their father suffered from a chronic involutional melancholia with bizarre hypochondriacal delusions. Slater thought the most reasonable explanation was that all three members of the family suffered from a schizophrenic psychosis in which a depressive factor played a prominent role. The case histories and Slater's discussion and analysis of them remain as valuable as ever as examples of good psychiatric observation and reporting, and perceptive comments.

Today research is more complex. There are aspects of Slater's classic study that would be questioned if they were put forward in a research application now, some 40 years later. A referee might complain that the diagnostic criteria were nowhere specifically stated. There was no attempt to assess their reliability. Nurses were not asked to complete behaviour rating scales. The principal and only investigator was to decide whether a pair was MZ or DZ and make the psychiatric diagnosis of both twins.

How far failure to meet such objections might have biased the results in this study has been discussed at length elsewhere (Rosenthal, 1962; Gottesman and Shields, 1966) and is old history now. On the question of contaminated diagnosis, Slater may have allowed himself to be influenced by the proband's diagnosis as well as by the history of the co-twin in classifying some clearly abnormal co-twin where, as inevitably in a systematically ascertained sample, information was inadequate; but the uncertainties are always made explicit (e.g. Case 67, p. 143, where the co-twin is listed as suicide, ?schizophrenia, on the evidence of his unexpectedly studying books on medicines and poisons, a lack of concern about his twin's illness and lying late in bed in the mornings). There were also cases among the discordant pairs where a possibility of schizophrenia arose; but, there being less convincing evidence of psychosis, a different classification of the co-twin was made (e.g. Case 133, p. 181, psychopath). I know no example of Slater having changed a diagnosis to fit a theory. In Case 11 he did not re-diagnose the father as a schizophrenic; he remains in the analysis of results as having an affective disorder. Case 2 remains an example of schizophrenia in one twin and (reactive) depression in the other. I do not suppose the idea ever occurred to Slater that he might re-diagnose the proband as depressive, transfer her to the affective group and call the pair concordant! As he put it himself in his 'Auto-biographical sketch' (1971) in *Man, Mind, and Heredity* (p. 18) 'These were the days before anyone thought of a double-blind diagnosis, and the only way to scientific integrity was to set the standard of evidence for a firm diagnosis, and for a "probable" diagnosis, and try to abide by them consistently, even when one saw the evidence going against the working hypothesis'.

Slater's 1935 twin study included affective illness, organic states and neurotic or personality disorders as well as schizophrenia. While schizophrenia occurred most frequently in the families of schizophrenics, affective illness in the families of the manic-depressives and so on, this was very far from being exclusively the case. It is perhaps not surprising that in some studies today a still greater diagnostic mixture in families is reported. One can even find reports that 26.6 per cent of the children of manic-depressives are schizophrenic (Cammer, 1970) and that only 1.7 per cent of the first-degree relatives of affective psychotics are manic-depressives, whereas 15 per cent are schizophrenic (Reed, *et al,* 1973). At some centres one may suspect an over-diagnosis of schizophrenia. However, attempts to apply strict diagnostic criteria could also lead to failure to detect any family resemblance that might exist. If before the war the psychiatric hospitals in Slater's experience tended to under-diagnose schizophrenia, in the 1960s some hospitals may have over-diagnosed it. In Tsuang's (1967) study of pairs of hospitalized sibs, Slater diagnosed schizophrenia less often than the hospital psychiatrists. Diagnosing summaries of the histories blind, he failed to find significant resemblance between the sibs so far as schizophrenia was concerned. The final hospital diagnosis however—and even more so a diagnosis of schizophrenia made at any time—did indicate a significant resemblance. The relative failure of Slater's stricter requirements may have resulted from the fact that the clinical notes were not written up in sufficient detail for the purpose, or that it had not been possible to follow up both sibs. Tsuang's paper went on to show that there were several sib pairs where, as in the earlier twin study, illnesses were similar even though they received different diagnoses.

In the more recent Maudsley schizophrenic twin study (Gottesman and Shields, 1972) we experimented with multiple international blind diagnosis of the twins. Slater was the first of our judges. Among the six on whose judgements a consensus diagnosis was reached it is appropriate that as author of a leading textbook (Slater and Roth, 1969) Slater's usage of schizophrenia, with and without the inclusion of ?schizophrenia, was third or fourth in order of frequency; and he was most often in agreement with the other judges. As a rule, Slater would only make the diagnosis if there was a record of characteristically schizophrenic phenomena of a delusional or a hallucinatory kind. There were occasional exceptions, however, as in Case MZ 11A ('atypical benign schizophrenia') where he gave weight to the fact that all doctors who had seen the patient when ill had unhesitatingly considered him to be schizophrenic. It had long been my hope that in this study we would be able to obtain from him not only a blind diagnosis in accordance with modern research practice, but also the diagnosis he might have given had he been carrying out the study himself on the same lines as his earlier report. We therefore invited him to review four MZ pairs in which he had disagreed with the consensus diagnosis of schizophrenia or ?schizophrenia in one of the twins. His blind diagnoses had been:

Pair No.	Twin A	Twin B
6	Catatonic schizophrenia	Endogenous depression, inadequate personality
13	Inadequate personality	Schizo-affective (atypical)
15	Inadequate personality	Paranoid schizophrenia
23	Acute paranoid schizophrenia	Schizoid personality, ?insidious schizophrenia

He was provided with the complete abstract of the hospital notes and full transcript of the tape-recorded follow-up interview for both twins. In the first three pairs he concluded that schizophrenia was much the most likely diagnosis for both twins. A typical comment (Pair 6): 'It seems impossible to think that B's very similar illness, also leading to partial invalidism, is anything else than schizophrenia too'. Certainly neither Pair 6 nor Pair 13 would be a convincing example of schizophrenia in one twin and manic-depressive psychosis in the other. While there are obvious advantages in the objectivity of having diagnoses made blind, there are also similarities and differences in twins which can be obscured by this procedure. There are advantages in a clinical approach too.

In the fourth pair (23), Slater was impressed by the similar personality development of the two twins, but he did not wish to change his earlier diagnoses. He continued to count the pair as discordant, at least at present. 'There can be no reasonable doubt', he said, 'that A had a psychotic illness. The fact that he did, to my mind, does not much alter the probabilities in the case of his twin. The relevance of knowledge of one twin's illness to the problem of diagnosis in the other affects only quality not degree of abnormal state'. This well illustrates the point made above concerning the diagnosis of the co-twins in Slater's own study.

Slater's 'unblindfolded' diagnoses would have resulted in an MZ concordance rate in the Maudsley study only about 7 per cent lower than the one he obtained in his early study based on LCC mental hospital probands. Using the proband method the uncorrected concordance rate might have been 61 per cent compared with 68 per cent.

If, as I have suggested, Slater avoided any tendency to change diagnoses to fit a theory, he did change his theories in the light of his diagnoses. This happened when we followed up twins treated at the Maudsley and diagnosed as 'hysteria'. In the Retrospect (1971) which he contributed to his *Selected Papers* he wrote (p. 376):

> I confidently expected that positive concordances would emerge, higher in the MZ than in the DZ pairs. When quite different results came in . . . I can remember feeling very perplexed. New ideas had to be taken into account; and I had to think the thing through from the ground up, to the point where I doubted the very existence of a hysterical syndrome (or reaction type, or personality type). It was painful. It meant I had to go back on ideas I had published, and had, for instance, to re-write a section on 'hysteria' in the textbook . . . it was a *volte face* as uncomfortable and as invigorating as when a growing acquaintance with German phenomenological teaching drove me out of the comfortable school of Adolf Meyer.

What happened (Slater, 1961) was that none of twelve MZ or twelve DZ co-twins had ever received a diagnosis of hysteria;[*] abnormalities of one kind or another were about as common in the DZ and the MZ partners; and the probands' hysterical symptomatology was considered on follow-up to have most likely been secondary to some other condition. The most likely diagnoses of the 24 probands were thought to have been:

---

[*] We have subsequently found one concordant male MZ pair among some 700 twins referred to the Maudsley Hospital!

8 psychopaths (usually described as 'mainly hysterical');
4 anxiety or tension states; 3 other neuroses (including a compensation neurosis in an anxious personality);
3 cases of endogenous depression or cyclothymia;
1 schizophrenia; and 5 cases of epilepsy or other organic brain disorder (including a temporal abscess diagnosed post-mortem in a woman consistently classified as hysterical).

Some of these diagnoses, such as the schizophrenia and the temporal lobe abscess, were entirely secure. Slater's seeing an 'hysterical' episode in a manic-depressive family (DZ 9) makes excellent sense—at least to those with similar views about that disorder. But some of the diagnoses are admittedly more conjectural. One should not expect all the depressives or epileptics to be acceptable as probands in a study based on prototypic cases.

One of the more speculative proband diagnoses was that of DZ 12 where Slater suggested a physical basis, possibly a lesion of the paracentral lobule. Eight years after the 1960 follow-up the patient was seen again as a Maudsley outpatient with complaints related to the vision of the left eye. No abnormal physical signs could be found any more than they could when she had presented previously with left-sided symptoms similar to a stroke, but her complaints were reminiscent of those associated with chronic glaucoma. There was no longer any mention of the increased libido which had given rise to suspicions of a lesion. There had, however, been a recent hospital admission for depression for which ECT had been given. Instead of diagnosing hysteria the Maudsley consultant (now Dr Denis Leigh) recorded 'diagnosis uncertain', the likelihood lying between glaucoma and underlying depressive illness. Perhaps this can be seen as an influence of Slater's views on 'hysteria'.

The subsequent work on Maudsley neurotic and personality disordered twins in which Slater took part (Slater and Shields, 1969; Shields and Slater, 1971), was based on 192 probands who had received a non-psychotic, non-organic diagnosis at the Maudsley Hospital between 1948 and 1958. This time the follow-up diagnoses were made by Slater from summaries which did not mention the zygosity or diagnosis of the other twin. Briefly, the findings suggested a genetic component in anxiety states and personality disorders but not in other neuroses (mostly reactive depressions). In a study of such dimensions it was impossible to give case histories as had been done in the schizophrenia and hysteria studies. A few comments on Slater's diagnostic practice may, therefore be appropriate here.

Maudsley index and Slater follow-up diagnoses of the probands, made seven and a half years later on average, differed considerably, as can be seen from Table 1. Indeed, they were less alike

TABLE I

Diagnoses (6th edn ICD Code) of probands at Maudsley Index Admission and by Slater at follow-up

	Maudsley diagnosis			
	310–318	320–326		
		personality	other	
	neurosis	disorder	uncertain	Total
Slater's follow-up diagnosis:				
310–318 neurosis	75	1	2	78
320–326 personality disorder	32	34	2	68
300–309 psychosis	33	7	1	41
organic disorder	4	1	–	5
Total	144	43	5	192

than those of proband and MZ co-twin according to Slater. Of the 192 probands, 41 were now given a 'psychotic' diagnostic code—25 endogenous affective disorder, 13 schizophrenia and 3 organic psychosis. Five were diagnosed as having epilepsy or some other organic disorder. Many of these changes were the consequences of developments during the follow-up period. Within the groups of neurosis and personality disorder Slater used the latter classification more often than did the original Maudsley consultant. Thirty-two patients were moved by Slater from a neurotic to a personality disorder ICD code. He probably gave more weight both to previous personality and to subsequent course. Among the neuroses (78) Slater restricted his usage mainly to anxiety state (45) and reactive depression (24). There was good agreement over the anxiety states. Of 17 MZ probands so diagnosed by Slater 13 had previously received this diagnosis, 2 'phobias', 1 'obsessional neurosis' and 1 'hysteria'.

About half of the 68 'disorders of character, etc.' were coded by Slater as '320.3, pathological personality, inadequate' for want of a better category in the then current 6th edition of the ICD, but he usually specified the nature of the 'inadequacy'. It is interesting that in the eleven MZ pairs where both twins had a primary diagnosis of personality disorder the classification tended to be very similar in about half—e.g. both twins 'hysterical and cyclothymic mainly' or 'asocial, delinquent', or 'mainly anxious', while in others the diagnoses might be 'inadequate, obsessional symptomatology' in one twin and 'inadequate, mainly anxious and hypochondriacal' in the other.

Unfortunately there is nothing useful that can be said shortly from this study about the effect of Slater's usage of the 'endogenous depression' diagnosis. While he employed this more frequently than the Maudsley psychiatrists of the time (mostly before the advent of the antidepressants) he did so less frequently than Dr da Fonseca in some of the same cases.

A finding of considerable interest was the lack of any evidence for a genetic influence on reactive as opposed to endogenous depression. Reactive depression turned out to be more like hysteria so far as twin concordance rates were concerned. This may be largely because of the diagnostic criteria. Patients with recurrent episodes of depression or with abnormal personalities were not usually diagnosed as reactive depression. Studies of 'non-endogenous depression' in twins on the Danish twin register (Shapiro, 1970) and of neurotic twins seen in a Berlin clinic by a psychoanalyst (Schepank, 1974) suggest that genetic factors, though not so specific as those influencing manic-depressive psychosis, influence neurotic depression too. However, the differences in concordance rate between the studies are probably more apparent than real and depend on how personality disorder had been dealt with. Furthermore, numbers are small; even with 192 probands to start with we had only eight MZ pairs with a reactive depressive proband.

It is reassuring both for the investigator and for his scientific critics when positive findings in a clinical genetic study can be shown not to have arisen through the diagnostician's knowledge of the diagnosis of a close relative. This source of bias is excluded in our recent studies and it is gratifying that Slater's diagnostic acumen was still able to produce significant findings.

However, the diagnoses were made from summaries. I had prepared the summaries and I had seen or knew about both the twins. There are, I believe, advantages as well as disadvantages in the direct comparison of twins with one another, and it was hoped that the precautions taken were sufficient to avoid some of the disadvantages. But I also knew something of Slater's diagnostic practice. It could be argued that by selecting in a biased manner what I put in the summaries I could have influenced the results in such a way as to undo all the advantages of the supposed independent diagnosis of the twins and make a mockery of the whole procedure. However, I tried to follow the example of Slater himself when he prepared summaries for his earlier study, and in my own work I had been as much interested in differences as in similarities between twins. One of our principal aims when we set up the Maudsley Hospital Twin Register (Shields, 1968) was to obtain useful leads as to the environmental causes of the neuroses. In the summaries I always included the symptomatology in some detail and recorded all diagnostic opinions expressed. Since Slater's diagnoses often differed from those of the other psychiatrists in this study, this could not have been a cause for the degree of diagnostic concordance found in MZ pairs. It is also worth pointing out that Slater's concept of what is within normal limits is a tolerant one. Close to half the MZ co-twins were regarded as normal. Whether psychiatric help had been required or not carried weight with him in deciding whether or not a formal diagnosis was merited. For instance, 'complained of constipation' would not be diagnosed as 'probably obsessional neurosis', making a pair concordant for that diagnosis.

A final point on the question whether the procedure was sufficiently blind: the specific findings concerning anxiety neurosis, other neuroses and personality disorder were not predicted by me and are unlikely to have arisen because of the way I prepared the summaries. While it seemed clear as time went on that MZ twins would be found to be somewhat more concordant than DZ twins, I thought that diagnostic distinctions between, say, 'reactive depression (in a somewhat abnormal personality)' and 'personality disorder (liable to depression under minor stress)' might prove too unreliable for the separate diagnoses to show different patterns of concordance in a clinical genetic study. It remains to be seen whether our findings hold up in the hands of a less skilled diagnostician or the digits of a computer.

In my contribution to this volume I have commented on some of the diagnostic aspects of the twin studies on which Dr Slater and I have worked together. A primary aim was of course to evaluate the roles of genetic and environmental factors in the common but aetiologically obscure psychiaric disorders. But genetic studies can also be used to throw light on problems of psychiatric nosology. Family histories can be relevant in deciding how far we consider Huntington's chorea, bipolar psychosis and hysteria to be diseases and in elucidating the biological relationship of personality to mental illness. Such questions have arisen in other studies by Slater, usually without his having to make any diagnoses himself. One can mention his integrative, multidimensional theory of the neurotic constitution (Slater and Slater, 1944), based on his work at Sutton Emergency Hospital during the war; his monogenic theory of schizophrenia (Slater, 1958; Slater and Cowie, 1971), based on selected or pooled studies from the literature—another integrative theory; and his study of the schizophrenia-like psychoses of epilepsy (Slater, Beard and Glithero, 1963), carried out from the National Hospital, Queen Square, in which a small group of symptomatic schizophrenics was separated out from the main group, partly on the basis of their lack of a 'family history'.

After a period when the value of diagnosis in psychiatry was seriously questioned, increasing attention is nowadays paid to its uses and to improving its reliability. Old perennials such as the classification of the depressions and the breadth of heterogeneity of schizophrenia crop up again in new lights. Genetic studies will remain one method of seeking new solutions. Unfortunately for pedigree studies and for the follow-up of high-risk children a generation later, changes in diagnostic practices and in the most favoured ancillary tests mean that even the better recorded medical notes and research projects of one era are found to be unsuitable by investigators of the next. Slater found it impossible to reach even a probable diagnosis from the hospital records of the turn of the century when in about 1950 he attempted to analyse some of the data collected in Sir Frederick Mott's index of familial cases treated in the London County Council mental hospitals. He would be the first to admit that future generations will have their own—one hopes improved—methods and will find inadequacies from their point of view in even the best recorded histories in his twin studies. However, the studies I have mentioned are not yet of the ancient past, and for some time to come it should still be possible to learn from the way in which one clinician and scientist—Eliot Slater— dealt with the diagnostic problems.

References

Cammer, L. (1970) Schizophrenic children of manic-depressive parents. *Diseases of the Nervous System,* **31,** 177–80.

Gottesman, I. I. and Shields, J. (1966) Contributions of twin studies to perspectives on schizophrenia. In: *Progress in Experimental Personality Research,* vol. 3 (ed. B. A. Maher), New York: Academic Press, 1–84.

Gottesman, I. I. and Shields, J. (1972) *Schizophrenia and Genetics: a Twin Study Vantage Point.* New York: Academic Press.

Reed, S. C., Hartley, C., Anderson, V. E., Phillips, V. P. and Johnson, N. A. (1973) *The Psychoses: Family Studies.* Philadelphia, London, Toronto: Saunders.

Rosenthal, D. (1962) Problems of sampling and diagnosis in the major twin studies of schizophrenia. *Journal of Psychiatric Research,* **1,** 116–34.

Schepank, H. (1974) *Erb- und Umweltfaktoren bei Neurosen. Tiefenpsychologische Untersuchungen an 50 Zwillingspaaren.* Monographien aus dem Gesamtgebiete der Psychiatrie, Psychiatry Series, Band 11. New York, Berlin, Heidelberg: Springer-Verlag.

Shapiro, R. W. (1970) A twin study of non-endogenous depression. *Acta Jutlandica,* **42** (2).

Shields, J. (1968) Psychiatric genetics. In: *Studies in Psychiatry* (ed. M. Shepherd and D. L. Davies). London: Oxford University Press, 169–91.

Shields, J. and Gottesman, I. I. (1972) Cross-national diagnosis of schizophrenia in twins. *Archives of General Psychiatry,* **27,** 725–30.

Shields, J. and Slater, E. (1971) Diagnostic similarity in twins with neuroses and personality disorders. In: *Man, Mind, and Heredity: Selected Papers of Eliot Slater on Psychiatry and Genetics* (ed. J. Shields and I. I. Gottesman). Baltimore and London: Johns Hopkins Press, 252–7. (First published in French in *L'Évolution Psychiatrique,* **31,** 441–51 (1966).)

Slater, E. (with the assistance of J. Shields) (1953) *Psychotic and Neurotic Illnesses in Twins*. Medical Research Council Special Report Series No. 278, London: Her Majesty's Stationery Office.

Slater, E. (1958) The monogenic theory of schizophrenia. *Acta Genetica Statistica et Medica*, **8**, 50–6.

Slater, E. (1961) The thirty-fifth Maudsley Lecture: 'Hysteria 311'. *Journal of Mental Science*, **107**, 359–81.

Slater, E. (1971) Autobiographical Sketch, and Retrospect. In: *Man, Mind, and Heredity: Selected Papers of Eliot Slater on Psychiatry and Genetics* (ed. J. Shields and I. I. Gottesman). Baltimore and London: Johns Hopkins Press, 1–23 and 367–80.

Slater, E., Beard A. W. and Glithero, E. (1963) The schizophrenia-like psychoses of epilepsy. *British Journal of Psychiatry*, **109**, 95–150.

Slater, E. and Cowie, V. A. (1971) *The Genetics of Mental Disorders*. London: Oxford University Press.

Slater, E. and Roth, M. (1969) *Mayer-Gross, Slater and Roth Clinical Psychiatry*, 3rd edn. London: Baillière, Tindall and Cassell.

Slater, and Shields, J. (1969) Genetical aspects of anxiety. In: *Studies of Anxiety* (ed. M. H. Lader). British Journal of Psychiatry Special Publication No. 3. Ashford, Kent: Headley, 62–71.

Slater, E. and Slater, P. (1944) A heuristic theory of neurosis. *Journal of Neurology and Psychiatry*, **7**, 49–55.

Tsuang, M-t. (1967) A study of pairs of sibs both hospitalized for mental disorder. *British Journal of Psychiatry*, **113**, 283–300.

ASPECTS OF CONTINUITY IN THE AETIOLOGY OF MENTAL DISORDER

Erik Essen-Möller

In honour of Eliot Slater I should like to set out here some various opinions on continuity and discontinuity within psychiatry, a subject with which Eliot Slater concerned himself, directly or indirectly, in connection with a number of different themes. This topic also provides an opportunity for presenting to English-speaking colleagues certain ideas of a Swedish psychiatrist, the late Professor Henrik Sjöbring (1879–1956), who was my teacher. Although his work is as yet little known outside Sweden, it roused Eliot Slater's interest, and they met.

Continuous variation in personality

Sjöbring suggested that in the century (posthumous work, 1973) the endless continuity of personality variants which it seems impossible to map might be composed of a limited number of independent dimensions of variation, each of them displaying approximately a Gaussian distribution. However, with the exception of variation in intelligence, the bearings of the postulated dimensions were so far unknown.

For a dimension to have biological relevance, in Sjöbring's view it ought to be developmental in nature. Thus an individual's position on such a scale would indicate how far he was able to develop or adapt in that particular direction by virtue of genetic predisposition, most people stopping midway and minorities either leading or lagging behind. Accordingly Sjöbring considered the left tail variants of each such dimension to be less developed or adaptable, and therefore likely to be over-represented among patients with a functional mental disorder. Independently of Sjöbring, this was also what Slater thought when he used his clinical data for building his multidimensional genetic model of personality variation (1943,

45

1944, 1950a). Sjöbring, who had started from the multivariate concept, saw rather a chance of identifying some of the dimensions clinically and theoretically.

Pierre Janet (1894, 1898, 1903, 1909) and Eduard Reiss (1910) had at that time described three types of personality each of which apparently predisposed to a different type of functional decompensation: asthenic-obsessive, hysteric-primitive, and manic-depressive respectively. Sjöbring ventured to suggest that these might represent left tail variants in the developmental sense. If so, the various traits to be found with each type of personality would largely reflect a single basic character. Janet had already suggested explanations to this effect. Sjöbring worked them out so as to fit a wider psychological model.

Indeed Sjöbring had also engaged in outlining a general model of mental functioning and its perpetual development, at a formal and elemental level. For this endeavour he sought inspiration from the works of Theodor Lipps (1902–1907). The model was a fascinating construct that brought together cognitive, conative and emotional aspects into a single view, as sides of the same psychological process. It suggested, for instance, how traits like coolness and propensity for abstraction were connected, and how the same event or perception could elicit different emotional responses according to the individual's earlier experience. What Sjöbring presented here was in fact a theory of emotions much his own, based on a principle of elemental biodynamic development and continuity. It will not be possible here to expand on this matter.

It was into this general model, however, that Sjöbring fitted the three characters which he held basic to the left tail variants mentioned, and so a clue had been found for defining tentatively three developmental dimensions of personality with regard to their formal nature. The corresponding right tail variants were then inferred, and identified in the population. Sjöbring called his dimensions validity, solidity and stability. Intelligence, or capacity, was seen as a similar dimension. There are some striking analogies with Pavlovian typology (1935), and relations to certain other systems of personality variation were discussed by Nyman (1956).

In spite of their hypothetical nature, Sjöbring's continuous developmental dimensions proved very useful in clinical work, taking regard of assets and weaknesses alike. They are thoroughly described in his posthumous work (1973). Questionnaires for self-rating were constructed by Marke and Nyman (MNT, 1962) and independently by Bagge (1963). The MNT scale was also published in Italian by Perris (1970) and in English by Coppen (1966), Barrett, (1972), Metcalfe *et al* (1975), and Johnson *et al* (1975). Nyman (1956) gave some instances of behavioural rating, a kind of observation favoured by Sjöbring himself. Presentations, discussions and applications of Sjöbring's ideas were listed by Essen-Möller (1977b).

Discontinuous variation due to lesions

Severe mental defects, as we know, are sometimes due to early brain injury. Obviously, in spite of their being measured on the same descriptive scale of intelligence quotients, they are *not* continuous with natural intelligence variation from a biological point of view. This dichotomy into 'lesional' and 'natural' was also applied by Sjöbring to personality variation.

Unlike the ubiquitous natural variants, to which belong the developmental variants mentioned in the preceding section, lesions occur in a limited number of persons. To use a formulation of Sjöbring's, a lesion either retards the development that would otherwise have been natural for the person in question or makes it deviate from its course. Since this is also the effect of abnormal genes, Sjöbring used to include them with his concept of lesions. After all, a genetic mutation might be seen as reflecting an early lesion.

As long as the lesion is mild or moderate, the natural variants of the personality may still dominate the picture or at least remain perceptible. Therefore an apparent continuity from severely abnormal to entirely normal, such as is suggested by Kretschner (1921) and E. Bleuler (1922) for the variation from schizophrenic to schizothymic, and by Schneider (1923) for the psychopathic personalities, might be deceptive and due to a confusion of the two kinds of variation. A more or less severe abnormality might have been superimposed upon natural variants consisting of different combinations and shadings of normal qualities in the personality (Essen-Möller, 1946; Nyman, 1955).

To appreciate the lesional variants it will be necessary to be familiar with the natural; the converse is also true. Discrimination will at times be difficult, but this should not be allowed to blur the principal distinction between the two kinds of variants.

When Sjöbring first built up his view of the developmental variants, he started from personalities associated with functional disorders exclusively, and even the premorbid traits to be seen in many schizophrenics were left out of consideration. In this way he intended to guard himself from an admixture of lesional factors. It was only much later, when confronted with the many mild functional disorders that were seen in the psychiatric unit of a teaching hospital, that Sjöbring began to suspect that lesional factors might play a far greater role than he had imagined. Quite frequently a 'neurosis' seemed to have been caused by some physical illness, not least a viral or other infection. Where situational stress was the precipitant, it was often in a person already weakened by a physical ailment, dating back perhaps to earlier years. It was noteworthy that among Slater's soldiers those who broke down following only a minimal stress frequently showed signs of poor physical health, having histories of illness including chronic bronchitis and rheumatic infections (1950b).

Once Sjöbring had perceived the role of lesions in general, it sometimes happened that he surprised his pupils by accepting a lesional aetiology as plausible even when the mental decompensation appeared to precede it. Thus in a certain case where an inexplicable, longstanding depression in a healthy young person was complicated after a couple of months by irritability and hypersensitivity to noise, and later still herpes zoster, Sjöbring suggested that a subclinical viral infection had caused the depression. After all, his line of thought appeared reasonable. The banal paradigm of the order of events seeming to be reversed in this way is of course the well-behaved little child who is suddenly naughty and insufferable and the next day has a fever. Mothers rather than fathers will make the correct diagnosis!

However, to Sjöbring it was not only a matter of association in time. He studied with interest the nature of signs, for instance the longstanding anomalies of tonus and alertness that were frequent with Sydenham's chorea, the similar more ephemeral signs with the common cold or allergy, the hyperirritability that sometimes follows cerebral concussion. He made it routine to look for such signs, and was often able to demonstrate them convincingly. Of course inherited anomalies were also taken into consideration.

On the whole it can be said that the mild lesional traits by which Sjöbring was fascinated can be seen as slight forms of well-known organic syndromes. He was inclined to accept them in their own right, even where current methods of physical examination failed to reveal their origin. We should train ourselves to see the vestigial effusiveness that may appear as senescence supervenes, or as a first sign of inebriation, and be aware of the difference from natural warmth. We should learn to distinguish pathologic rigidity and stubbornness from natural consistency and firmness of character, and so on. For a clinical description of some lesional traits, see Sjöbring (1973), G. Uddenberg (1955), Essen-Möller et al (1956) and Kaij (1960).

In recognizing such mild lesional traits Sjöbring was aided by his habit of asking himself, in terms of himself, in terms of his general model of elemental mental functioning, about the significance of everything observed, and of course by comparing it with his notion of the developmental variants and the gross organic syndromes. Thus feeling his way from both sides, the natural and the lesional, he gradually adjusted his outlook. Indeed he ended up with the view that even those 'functional' illnesses and personality types from which he once had started his search for developmental variants mostly contained an added lesional component (Essen-Möller, 1943). His concept of the developmental variants became more pathoplastic than pathogenetic. He came to think that as a rule they show only moderate and transient reactions, with little need for psychiatric care unless the person has been exposed to quite extraordinary stresses.

It is difficult to judge to what extent Sjöbring may have exaggerated the role of the lesional. It may be of some relevance to note that the majority of his patients came from a rural area and a small university city, not from a big industrial town. In essence Sjöbring appears to have been before his time. The recent reports on minimal brain dysfunction syndromes are well known (Wender, 1972). Subtle electroencephalographic deviations are now known to occur more frequently in psychiatric populations than in controls (Frey and Steinwall 1953, Frey 1970). From Sjöbring's former department, Nilson and Smith (1962) reported a lower average alpha rhythm in a particular (chalarophrenic) type of personality described as lesional by Sjöbring. Uddenberg (1955) found prospectively an increased frequency of nervous manifestations in prematurely born children. A higher rate of first consultations for nervous complaints was also found prospectively in a non-clinical population among those who had previously been rated lesional according to Sjöbring's method (Magnell, 1966, Essen-Möller and Eagnell, 1975). If this does not prove that the traits observed were actually lesional, it still seems to indicate that some meaningful differentiation is possible even among socially healthy persons.

Genetic continuity and discontinuity

Continuous variation of normal traits, insofar as they are genetically determined, is often explained by a polygenic model. Here several genes belonging to different loci are assumed to work additively in the same direction. Since the effect of each of them is considered minute, and is also modified by other genes and by environment, no discernible segregation or discontinuity is to be expected. Theoretically this kind of variation had been studied under the assumption that the number of pertinent polygenes present in each individual is distributed approximately according to a Gaussian curve.

Between close relatives the amount of polygenes present will be positively correlated. In good concordance with this, Roberts (1952) demonstrated that the mean IQ of a sibship tends to increase or decrease with the IQ of its index cases as long as this remains within normal limits, down to and including the mildly retarded.

Interestingly, no such correlation was found in sibs of index cases with severe mental defect. Except for sporadic defectives, they gathered instead around the mean of the population at large. This can be taken to indicate that the defect was due to some abnormal factor, genetic or exogenic, which rather than forming part of the normal distribution had superimposed itself upon it randomly.

Morbid inheritance has long been considered monogenic (Lenz, 1927), that is to say, discontinuous. It is true that one has been aware of the possibility that this opinion was biased, since discontinuity is what lends itself most obviously to study. However, it is only recently that polygenic inheritance has been seriously considered as a possible explanation of certain morbid conditions, among them schizophrenia (Edwards, 1960, 1972; Gottesman and Shields, 1972). Here the assumption is that a limiting number of pertinent polygenes has to be present, a so-called threshold effect. (By the way, why is it that authors explaining the threshold phenomenon by means of diagrams insist on placing the morbid condition in the *right* tail of the distribution, suggesting more or less that it crowns development?)

The preference shown by several authors for the polygenic model partly stems from certain difficulties with the monogenic interpretation. For one thing, schizophrenia retains (or is believed to retain) its frequency in the population in spite of low fertility. Indeed the reproduction of classical schizophrenics is too low to be compensated by the ordinary rate of mutations at a single locus, and no reproductive advantage has so far been proven in non-schizophrenic relatives (although other advantage was suggested by Heston, 1966, Karlsson, 1970, and Farley, 1976). This difficulty was held to be by-passed if the required amount of mutations could be assumed to be delivered jointly by a multiplicity of polygenes. I do not feel, however, that the possibilities of explaining the constant frequency even on a monogenic model have been exhausted (Heston, 1970; Kidd, 1975).

Another alleged difficulty for the monogenic, preferably dominant, model of schizophrenia is the considerable gap between the observed and the expected (Mendelian) risk to close relatives of index cases, amounting to 10 per cent and 50 per cent respectively. The gap has been explained as being due to reduced penetrance of the gene in question; but this was considered by some an adhoc hypothesis that had better be avoided. Yet we can see from the 50 per cent discordance in monozygotic twins that considerable environmental influence is a reality. Between relatives other than monozygotic twins the environmental differences may be greater still and a variation due to differences in the total genetic constitution has to be added.

We may also choose to include certain other disorders and anomalies with the cases of classical schizophrenia among relatives, and regard them as incomplete manifestations of the abnormal gene. Admittedly the exact frequency of such 'spectrum disorders' is not known because of difficulties of definition, but I guess they may well outnumber the classical psychoses and cover a good deal of the gap (Lenz, 1937; Essen-Möller, 1941; Heston, 1970)—we should not, perhaps, expect to be able to cover it completely. The point is that a reduced penetrance or manifestation, whether graded or not, appears a justified and reasonable explanation for the deviance from monogenic Mendelian proportions.

Speaking of schizophrenic spectrum disorders, to my mind comprehensive terms like psychosis, neurosis, or psychopathic, sociopathic and even schizoid personality are of little use as definitions. Rather it should be possible to define within any such category, and also among socially healthy individuals, a number of indicative anomalies of a more elemental kind, e.g. with regard to accessibility, flexibility, concentration, facial tone (Essen-Möller, 1941), ways of thinking (Singer and Wynne, 1965), maybe eye-tracking (Holzman *et al,* 1974). Spectrum disorders were also discussed by Alanen (1966), Heston (1966), Rosenthal and van Dyke (1970), Rosenthal (1975), Planansky (1972), Cadoret (1973), Sedgwick (1973), Shields *et al* (1975), Kay *et al* (1975), Farley (1976), Nyman *et al* (1978) and Vanggaard (1978).

Of course it may seem inviting to interpret, as is sometimes done, the spectrum disorders as representing quantitative intermediates on a continuous polygenic load scale. On the other hand, there seems to be no compelling reason for abandoning the monogenic model on behalf of these disorders alone. And it would indeed be hard to agree on an order of sequence by which the diversified clinical pictures would plausibly reflect the subsumed variation in polygenic (cf Gottesman and Shields, 1971, p 520). Who decides whether a lack of concentration should be rated less severe, or more severe, than facial rigidity, a picture of obsessions, a tinge of suspiciousness in a non-schizophrenic relative? In our present state of ignorance, a designation like 'genetic circle' ('Erbkreis', Luxenburger, 1936) would appear perhaps more neutral, and less suggestive, than the linear 'spectrum'. And could we not quite as well, or even better, regard such various features as genetically equivalent? The action of a single morbid gene might well be different in different individuals, engaging perhaps different functional strucutures. Even Huntington's chorea, an agreed monogenic disease, has its spectrum disorders (Panse, 1942). And schizophrenic spectrum disorders occur in monozygotic co-twins of schizophrenics, where genetic differences are out of question.

A hypothesis put forward by Bleuler (1972) runs approximately as follows: (a) The functions engaged in schizophrenic illness, indeed the very personality, are so highly evolved and complex that they can hardly be imagined otherwise than as polygenically founded (cf Farley, 1976); (b) From a clinical point of view, schizophrenia represents a disharmony between intrinsically healthy functions, e.g. rational and irrational thinking occurring without mutual balance and in the wrong proportions; (c) Accordingly, in Bleuler's view, we should be dealing here with a disharmony between normal polygenes, brought together by unfortunate matings.

Against this view we may object that in every illness, according to the principle of Hughlings Jackson, the productive symptoms consist of intrinsically healthy functions which owing to some basic deficiency of disturbance have lost their regulation and mutual balance or harmony. Moreover, what we are striving to elucidate is the genetics of the disease, of the disturbance as such, not of the functions disturbed. In general with hereditary diseases it does not prove possible to infer from symptomatology alone how this basic disturbance is represented genetically.

Bleuler furthermore discusses whether the polygenes assumed to underlie schizophrenia are actually normal, or whether they should, after all, be regarded as abnormal. This is an interesting theoretical problem that may apply also to other illnesses, like diabetes and hypertension, for which the polygenic model has been considered. For the neurotic personalities, Slater (1942, 1944, 1950a) suggested an agglomeration of 'non-specific' (normal) polygenes. To me, as a pupil of Sjöbring, it appeared attractive to imagine, in such instances, an abnormal single gene which would then superimpose itself upon the normal polygenic personality or constitution (Essen-Möller, 1946, 1952). For the variation of intelligence, we have seen that a combined genetic model of this type is valid. Indeed Brown (1942) suggested it for the neuroses, and Slater (1947) applied it to certain intrafamilial variation in the detailed symptomatology of schizophrenia. I have mentioned that Lenz (1937) as well as Heston (1970) were of this opinion with regard to schizophrenia as a whole.

There is an evolutional aspect involved in this contrasting of normal and abnormal polygenes. In pursuit of a line of thought formulated by Medawar (1960, p 34) in a different context, one may ask how an agglomeration of abnormal polygenes could at all have come into being when the intermediate stages already display a reproductive fitness lower than average? We know that the average marriage rate is low in non-schizophrenic sibs of schizophrenics, presumably because of certain inherited characterological features displayed in some of them. Again it appears simpler to assume a single mutant gene for spectrum disorders and full-blown schizophrenia alike.

It is of great interest to note, in this connection, that adherents to the polygenic model of schizophrenia seem themselves to entertain some doubt. Some of them tentatively suggest that, out of the polygenes, one particular gene might be specific and requisite for the illness to appear. Granted the presence of this gene (not necessarily the same in all schizophrenic families), the remaining polygenes, together with environmental influences, would regulate the degree of penetrance and the clinical type of manifestation. Now this is precisely the model I have in mind, only I should much prefer to call it *mono*genic. To be sure, any major gene will act within the setting of other genes, that is to say the individual's entire genetic constitution; but this is hardly what should be meant by polygenic transmission of a disease.

Let us now proceed from general considerations to empiric family statistics. Experts state that polygenic- and monogenic-dominant models will often yield similar risks to relatives of index cases, a fact that made Edwards (1960) coin the expression 'simulation of Mendelism'. Yet certain possibilities for discrimination are left open.

Thus monogenic dominance, as we have seen, requires 50 per cent incidence in sibs of schizophrenics, while the empiric risk is around 10 per cent, leading to the hypothesis of reduced penetrance of the gene. On the polygenic model expectancy is actually 10 per cent so that the empiric finding hits the point. However, this apparent support for the polygenic model is invalidated by the fact that reduced penetrance has also to be allowed for here, considering the high rate of discordance in monozygotic twins (Shields and Slater, 1967). In other words, the empiric finding is far too high to fit the polygenic model.

Another possibility for discrimination would be that the expected risk to grandchildren and nephews–nieces amounts to half the risk to children and sibs on the dominant model but is lower on the polygenic. The actual risk is mostly reported to be low, thus seemingly in favour of the polygenic model. However, it is the healthier of the children and sibs who most frequently marry and transmit their genes to the next generation. This will lower the risk in both alternatives and probably will make it more difficult to establish a difference between them.

Slater and Tsuang (1968) made an inquiry into unilateral and bilateral taint, thus hoping to be able to discriminate between the two models. Unfortunately, however, the results did not reach significance in either direction.

Strömgen (1968, p 70) felt that the distribution of schizophrenics, deviant personalities and normals among the offspring of schizophrenic couples tends to bimodality, which then would argue against polygenic transmission.

Odegaard (1972) reported a positive correlation with regard to number of psychoses between different categories of relatives of the same index cases. This type of correlation should not occur with dominance, and at first sight I was inclined to accept it as indicative of polygenic inheritance, the opinion of Ödegaard himself. However, the finding could not be replicated in a sample of my own, maybe partly because my index cases were all schizophrenic while Ödegaard's consisted of patients with a functional psychosis and thus with mixed diagnoses (Essen-Möller, 1977a).

Other recent contributions to the discussion of mode of inheritance in schizophrenia are those of Kringlen (1967), Elston and Campbell (1970), Kay and Lindelius (1970), Slater and Cowie (171), Gottesman and Shields (1972), Dalén (1972), Karlsson (1974) and Cavelli-Sforza and Kidd (1975). For diseases in general, see also Morton (1967, p 30). It appears that a conclusive choice cannot be made today. Pending further evidence, however, the monogenic model strikes me personally as more verisimilar. So rather than subscribe to the suggested simulation of Mendelism, I look forward to its stimulation. Indeed the controversy is not merely academic. With a major gene there is the prospect of eventually discovering an enzymatic deficiency. And why not more than one? 'Schizophrenia' might represent a mixture of different diseases.

Before concluding this chapter, it remains to touch upon still another way of explaining a continuous variation genetically. I refer to the principle of multiple allelism, where a number of genes of different strength, all belonging to the same locus, build up a continuous variation by virtue of their pairwise combination. This is a somewhat different kind of monogenic model, and it appears easier here to imagine that extreme variants may be pathological. The model seems to have been introduced to psychiatry by Hoffmann (1922). It was extensively discussed by Conrad (1941), who used it for his own model of body-build and temperament variation, which was, incidentally, conceived as developmental in the same sense as the normal variants of Sjöbring. Indeed Sjöbring (1973, p 189) found the principle of multiple allelism compatible with his outlook, and he pointed out that even alternative traits, corresponding to the white and red flowers of Mendelian inheritance, might be explained on this model. Long ago (1943) I tried to suggest, perhaps inadequately, how the very rarity of extreme deviants in a multiple allelic system might cause their offspring to segregate, while the frequent individuals from the 'ordinary' part of the distribution would have their offspring differ only quantitatively. Unfortunately I have not come across any modern treatment of this problem.

Psychological continuity or understanding
A previously healthy young woman has, for the last few weeks, vomited every time she meets her mother. After negative physical examination she is referred to a psychiatric unit as a case of hysteria. In the ward she is seen to support herself against the wall of the corridor when in the company of nurses and patients, but she moves freely and gaily when not knowing herself observed. In spite of her behaviour, the psychiatrist in charge does not judge her a psychiatric case and sends her back for renewed neurological investigation. This is again negative, and once more she is referred to the psychiatric ward, where the idea of physical illness is still adhered to. She suddenly dies from cerebellar tumour.

Another case reported to me by a surgeon is the following. An adolescent boy, previously healthy and active if somewhat taciturn, was referred by his doctor for psychiatric observation since for a year or so he had refused working 'for no reason, by mere unwillingness'. He was soon dismissed for more thorough physical penetration, and this time was found to suffer from Krohn's disease, in urgent need of surgical treatment.

When these patients were referred from somaticists to psychiatrists, the diagnostic procedure appears to have been essentially one of elimination. As can be seen from Slater and Glithero's (1965) follow-up study of patients with a diagnosis of hysteria, it often happens that a psychological disorder is taken for granted where physical examination proves negative. I do not know whether some kind of psychological understanding has been attempted in the two cases mentioned; the symptom of vomiting might have been considered to convey the patient's unconscious hatred toward her mother.

Now why did the two psychiatrists in charge adhere to a notion of physical illness? Probably because they were not satisfied, for their part, that there was psychological continuity and understanding at a common-sense level. As we have seen, this was the direction of diagnostic elimination that proved correct in the examples offered.

Of course, errors occur in both directions, and actual psychological stresses may well escape notice even when severe (Ernst, 1956). On the other hand, successful unveiling of stresses and conflicts is not always equivalent to a solution of the aetiological problem, not even when therapeutically helpful.

Apart from mere coincidences and errors of recollection, there is a possibility that the patient himself was instrumental in building up the psychological situation which he subsequently came to experience as stressful. We may think of the well known discussion of this problem with regard to the over-protected children. Eberhard (1968) encountered the same problem in his registration of stress in monozygotic twins discordant for peptic ulcer. Bleuler (1972) dealt with it in his cautious evaluation of childhood stress in the histories of adult schizophrenics.

Psychological continuity and aetiology has been assumed where a schizophrenic was exposed as a child to the presence of schizophrenic relatives (Lidz, 1968). However, it appears that children who were adopted away from their schizophrenic families run much the same risk of falling ill (Heston, 1966; Rosenthal *et al,* 1968). Another indication of psychological continuity and aetiology has been seen in the fact that, among schizophrenic parents of schizophrenics, mothers outnumber the fathers (Alanen, 1958). However, this predominance of mothers turned out to be a retrospective statistical illusion (Essen-Möller, 1963), and seen prospectively the children of male and female schizophrenics run the same risk.

A stated continuity between events and reaction may prove to be limited to temporal sequence, or maybe to content, and still remain incomprehensible from the point of view of form or degree. Whence arose the hypersensitivity and irascibility? Whence came the particular intensity, the paranoid tinge, the propensity for psychodynamic complication? The fact that signs like these might strike as mere exaggerations of normal reactions certainly does not mean that they cannot be lesional in origin.

Aetiology should not be confounded with elicitation. We usually do not attribute the bursts of lachrymosity that can be seen in an arteriosclerotic patient to the grave tone of conversation by which he happened to be confronted. Doctors of the older generation will remember how the fidgetiness of young choreatic patients used to flourish at even minimal emotional stimulation, such as somebody entering the room. With some diseases of the basal ganglia veritable seizures of dystonic behaviour can be triggered by similarly banal disturbances. With our cerebellar patient the presence of her mother proved eliciting, and maybe the patient was particularly fond of her. But this was not the basic aetiology. Should we not make a habit of keeping such paradigms in mind when considering the aetiology of a common neurosis or other 'functional' disorder?

Is our patient, then, physically ill? Does he suffer a minor 'endogenous' change? Was he subjected at an earlier time to a persistent change in personality, following perhaps some physical illness or injury? Is there all the same a longstanding personality disorder to explain his way of reacting to the present situation? This indeed will be a frequent finding, but it should not mean the end of our search. Did the personality disorder, in its turn, date back to more distant experiences, or rather perhaps to some perinatal or prenatal lesion or even a genetic abnormality? At every level, opinions will differ.

Of course, these sketchy remarks on psychological understanding can hardly more than reflect from another angle the tenet of the preceding sections. In the aetiology of the mental disorders, even functional and mild, the doctrine of unbroken continuity and development should not be taken for granted.

Concluding remarks

Descriptive continuity from normal to abnormal personality and to neurotic and psychotic manifestations cannot always be regarded as indicative of a coresponding aetiologic continuity. For instance, the clinical existence of what has been called the schizophrenic spectrum disorders does not by itself enforce the adoption of a quantitative polygenic model of inheritance in schizophrenia. For other reasons also, and pending further evidence, one may well defend the older hypothesis of a single abnormal gene which is modified in its expression by the particular variant of (polygenic) personality or constitution upon which it happens to be grafted. This same idea of genetic discontinuity may also be thought to apply to many personality disorders and neuroses.

In a similar way superimposed upon normal variation is the effect of non-genetic lesions, the milder of which, though often overlooked, will reasonably be much more frequent than the severe ones with which we are generally familiar. Indeed the milder lesions might be thought to deliver another substantial part of the numerous mental disorders that are at present held to be genuinely psychological in origin. A lesion, like a genetic abnormality, may either produce the disorder over physical pathways exclusively, or may give rise to it indirectly through deflecting the development of the personality and its ways of reacting to psychological situations. These may then be mistaken for the ultimate cause.

Accumulating evidence from experimental and genetic studies as well as from retrospective and prospective investigations is today likely to make an increasing number of doctors conversant with this way of looking at things. The Swedish psychiatrist H. Sjöbring (1879–1956) arrived at it some 45 years ago by clinical observation alone. Strikingly, it was his interest in normal personality, its structure, development and inter-individual variation, that gradually led him to assign in the aetiology of the mild mental disorders a more primary role to medical factors and a more secondary to the psychological.

References

Alanen, Y. O. (1958) The mothers of schizophrenic patients. Diss. Helsinki, and *Acta psychiatrica et neurologica scandinavica, suppl. 124.*

Alanen, Y. O. (1966) The family in the pathogenesis of schizophrenic and neurotic disorders. *Acta psychiatrica scandinavica, suppl. 189.*

Bagge, L. (1963) *A Psychosomatic Approach to Cystic Glandular Hyperplasia of the Endometrium.* Diss. Lund. Uppsala: Almqvist and Wiksell.

Barrett, J. E. (1972) Use of the M-N-T inventory (Sjöbring personality dimensions) on an American population. *Acta psychiatrica scandinavica,* 48, 501–9.

Bleuler, E. (1922) Die Probleme der Schizoidie und der Zyntonie. *Zeitschrift für die gesamte Neurologie und Psychiatrie,* 78, 373–99.

Bleuler, M. (1972) *Die schizophrenen Geistesstörungen im Lichte langjährizer Kranken- und Familiengeschichten.* Stuttgart: Thieme.

Brown, F. W (1942) Heredity in the psychoneuroses. *Proceedings of the Royal Society of Medicine,* 35, 785–90.

Cadoret, K. J. (1973) Toward a definition of the schizoid state: evidence from studies of twins and their families. *British Journal of Psychiatry,* 122, 679–85.

Cavalli-Sforza, L. L. & Kidd, K. K. (1975) Genetic models for schizophrenia. *Neurosciences research program bulletin,* 10, 406–19.

Conrad, K. (1941) *Der Konstitutionstypus als genetisches Problem.* Berlin: Springer.

Coppen, A. (1966) The Merke–Nyman temperament scale, an English translation. *British Journal of Medical Psychology,* 39, 55–9.

Dalén, P. (1972) One, two, or many? *Genetic factors in 'schizophrenia'* (ed. A. R. Kaplan). Springfield: Thomas. 478–89.

Eberhard, G. (1968) Peptic ulcer in twins, a study in personality, heredity, and environment. Diss Lund, and *Acta psychiatrica scandinavica, suppl. 205.*

Edwards, J. H. (1960) The simulation of Mendelism. *Acta genetica statistica medica,* 10, 63–70.

Edwards, J. M. (1972) The genetical basis of schizophrenia. *Genetic factors in schizophrenia* (ed A. R. Kaplan). Springfield: Thomas, 311–14.

Elston, R. C. & Campbell, M. A. (1970) Schizophrenia: evidence for the major gene hypothesis. *Behaviour genetics,* 1, 3–10.

Ernst, K. (1956) 'Geordnete Familienverhältnisse' späterer Schizophrener in Lichte einer Nachuntersuchung. *Archiv für Psychiatrie und Nervenkrankheiten,* 194, 258–71.

Essen-Möller, E. (1941) Psychiatrische Untersuchungen an einer Serie von Zwillingen. *Acta psychiatrica et neurologica suppl. 23.*

Essen-Möller, E. (1943) Über den Begriff des Funktionellen und Organischen in der Psychiatrie. *Acta psychiatrica et neurologica,* 18, 1–44.

Essen-Möller, E. (1946) The concept of schizoidia. *Monthly review of psychiatry and neurology,* 112, 258–71.

Essen-Möller, E. (1952) La génétique dans la psychiatrie. *I er congrès international de psychiatrie en Paris 1950, comptes rendus des séances,* Vol. VI 79–84.

Essen-Möller, E. (1963) Über die Schizophreniehäufigkeit bei Müttern von Schizophrenen. *Schweizerisches Archiv für Neurologie, Neurochirurgie und Psychiatrie,* 91, 260–6.

Essen-Möller, E. (1977a) Evidence for polygenic transmission of schizophrenia? *Acta psychiatrica scandinavica,* 55, 202–7.

Essen-Möller, E. (1977b) A Sjöbring bibliography. *Nordisk psykiatrisk tidsskrift,* 31, 323-38.

Essen-Möller, E. and Hagnell, O (1975) 'Normal' and 'lesional' traits of personality according to Sjöbring: re-ratings and prognostic implications. *Neuropsychobiology,* 1, 146–54.

Essen-Möller, E. Larsson, M., Uddenberg, C. E. & White, G. (1956) Individual traits and morbidity in a Swedish rural population. *Acta psychiatrica et neurologica scandinavica, suppl. 100.*

Farley, J. D. (1976) Phylogenetic adaptations and the genetics of psychosis. *Acta psychiatrica scandinavica,* 53, 173–92.

Frey, T. S. (1970) Electroencephalographic alpha frequency and mental disease. *Acta psychiatrica scandinavica, suppl. 219,* 67–75.

Frey, T. S. & Steinwall, O. (1953) The electroencephalogram in minor psychiatric disorders. *Acta psychiatrica et neurologica scandinavica, suppl. 80.*

Gottesman, I. I. & Shields, J. (1971) Schizophrenia: geneticism and environmentalism. *Human Heredity,* 21, 517–22.

Gottesman, I. I. & Shields, J. (1972) *Schizophrenia and genetics, a twin study vantage point.* New York and London: Academic Press.

Hagnell, O (1966) *A Prospective Study of the Incidence of Mental Disorder.* Diss. Lund, Stockholm: Norstedts.

Heston, L. L. (1966) Psychiatric disorders in foster home reared children of schizophrenic mothers. *British Journal of Psychiatry,* 112, 819–25.

Heston, L. L. (1970) The genetics of schizophrenic and schizoid disease. *Science,* 16, 249–56.

Hoffmann, H. H. (1922) *Die individuelle Entwicklungskurve des Menschen, ein Problem der Konstitutions- und Vererbungslehre.* Berlin: Springer.

Holzman, P. S., Proctor, L. R., Levy, D. L., Yasillo, N. J., Meltzer, H. Y. & Hurt, S. W. (1974) Eye-tracking dysfunctions in schizophrenic patients and their relatives. *Archives of general psychiatry,* 31, 143–51.

Janet, P. (1894) *L'état mental des hystériques.* Paris: Rueff.

Janet, P. (1898) *Neuroses et idées fixes.* Paris: Alcan.

Janet, P. (1903) *Les obsessions et la psychasthénie.* Paris: Alcan.

Janet, P. (1909) *Les névroses.* Paris: Flammarion.

Johnson, A. L., Metcalfe, M. & Coppen, A. (1975) An analysis of the Marke–Nyman temperament scale. *British Journal of Social and Clinical Psychology,* 14, 379–85.

Kaij, L. (1960) *Alcoholism in Twins. Studies on the Etiology and Sequels of Abuse of Alcohol.* Diss Lund. Stockholm: Almqvist and Wiksell.

Karlsson, J. L. (1970) Genetic association of giftedness and creativity with schizophrenia. *Hereditas,* 66, 177–82.

Karlsson, J. L. (1974) Inheritance of schizophrenia. *Acta psychiatrica scandinavica, suppl. 247.*

Kay, D. W. K. & Lindelius, R., see Lindelius (1970).

Kay, D. K. W., Atkinson, M. W., Stephens, D. A., Rith, M. & Garside, R. F. (1975) Genetic hypotheses and environmental factors in the light of psychiatric morbidity in the families of schizophrenics. *British Journal of Psychiatry,* 127, 109–18.

Kidd, K. K. (1975) On the possible magnitudes of selective forces maintaining schizophrenia in the population. *Genetic research in psychiatry* (ed R. R. Fieve, D. Rosenthal and H. Brill). Baltimore and London: Johns Hopkins Press, 135–45.

Kretschmer, E. (1921) *Körperbau und Charakter.* Berlin: Springer.

Kringlen, E. (1967) *Heredity and Environment in the Functional Psychoses.* Diss. Oslo. Oslo: Universitetsforlaget.

Lenz, F. (1927) Die Krankhaften Erbanlagen. *Menschliche Erblehre und Rassenhygiene, I* (ed E. Baur, E. Fischer, and F. Lenz). Munich: Lehmann.

Lenz, F. (1937) Mendeln die Geisteskrankheiten? *Zeitschrift für induktive Abstammungs und Vererbungslehre,* 73, 559–71.

Lidz, Th. (1968) The family, language, and the transmission of schizophrenia. In *The Transmission of schizophrenia* (ed D. Rosenthal and S. S. Kety). Oxford and New York: Pergamon Press.

Lindelius, R. (ed) (1970) A study of schizophrenia. A clinical, prognostic and family investigation. *Acta psychiatrica scandinavica suppl. 216.*

Lipps, Th. (1902–1907) *Von Fühlen, Wollen und Denken.* Leipzig: Engelmann.

Lipps, Th. (1906) *Leitfaden der Psychologie.* Leipzig: Engelmann.

Luxenburger, H. (1936) Der heutige Stand der empirischen Erbprognose in der Psychiatrie als Grundlage für Massnahmen der Praktischen Gesundheitspflege. *Zentralblatt der Neurologie und Psychiatrie,* **81,** 12.

Marke, S. & Nyman, G. E. (1962) *Manual till MNT-skalan.* Stockholm: Svenska Testförlaget.

Medawar, P. B. (1960) *The Future of Man.* London: Methuen.

Metcalfe, M., Johnson, A. L. & Coppen, A. (1975) The Marke–Nyman temperament scale in depression. *British Journal of Psychiatry,* **126,** 41–8.

Morton, N. E. (1967) The detection of major genes under additive continuous variation. *American Journal of Human Genetics,* **19,** 22–34.

Nilsson, L. & Smith, G. J. W. (1962) Dimensions of overt behaviour as represented in EEG and adaptive test patterns. *Acta psychiatrica scandinavica,* **38,** 277–301.

Nyman, G. E. (1955) Typologische und dimensionale Anschauungen in der differentiellen Psychologie. *Anthrop. diff. et sci. typ. constit.* (Genève), **3,** 135–40.

Nyman, G. E. (1956) *Variations in personality.* Diss. Lund, and *Acta psychiatrica et neurologica, suppl. 70.*

Nyman, G. E., Nyman, K. & B. I. Nylander (1978) Non-regressive schizophrenia. *Acta psychiatrica scandinavica,* **57,** 165–92.

Ödegaard, Ö. (1972) The multifactorial theory of inheritance in predisposition to schizophrenia. In *Genetic Factors in 'Schizophrenia'* (ed A. R. Kaplan). Springfield: Thomas, 256–75.

Panse, F. (1942) *Die Erbchorea.* Leipzig: Thieme.

Pavlov, I. P. (1935) General types of animal and human higher nervous activity. *Selected Works.* Moscow: Foreign Languages Publication House, 315–44.

Perris, C. (1970) Scale Temperamentale di Marke e Nyman. Cremona.

Planansky, K. (1972) Phenotypic boundaries and genetic specificity in schizophrenia. *Genetic factors in 'Schizophrenia'* (ed A. R. Kaplan). Springfield: Thomas, 141–72.

Reiss, E. (1910) *Konstitutionelle Verstimmung und manisch-depressives Irresein.* Berlin: Springer.

Roberts, J. A. F. (1952) The genetics of mental deficiency. *Eugenics review,* **44,** 71–83.

Rosenthal, D. (1975) The concept of subschizophrenic disorders. In *Genetic Research in Psychiatry* (ed R. R. Fieve, D. Rosenthal and H. Brill). Baltimore and London: Johns Hopkins Press, 200–8.

Rosenthal, D. & van Dyke, J. (1970) The use of monozygotic twins discordant as to schizophrenia in the search for an inherited characterological defect *Acta psychiatrica scandinavica, suppl. 219,* 183–9.

Rosenthal, D., Wender, P. H., Kety, S. S., Schulsinger, F., Welner, J. & Östergaard, L. (1968) Schizophrenics' offspring reared in adoptive hopes, *The transmission of Schizophrenia* (ed D. Rosenthal and S. S. Kety). Oxford and New York: Pergamon Press 377–92.

Schneider, K. (1923) *Die psychopathischen Persönlichkeiten.* Vienna: Deuticke.

Sedgwick, P. (1973) The social analysis of schizophrenia. In *On the Origin of the Schizophrenic Psychoses* (ed H. M van Praag). Amsterdam: De Erven Bohn BV, 183–208.

Shields, J. & Slater, E. (1967) Genetic aspects of schizophrenia. *Hospital Medicine,* 579–84.

Shields, J., Heston, L. L. & Gottesman, I. I. (1975) Schizophrenia and the schizoid: a problem for genetic analysis. In *Genetic Research in Psychiatry* (ed R. R. Fieve, D. Rosenthal and H. Brill). Baltimore and London: Johns Hopkins Press, 167–97.

Singer, M. Th. & Wynne, L. C. (1965) Thought disorders and family relations of schizophrenics. *Archives of General Psychiatry*, 12, 187–212.

Sjöbring, H. (1973) Personality, structure and development, a model and its application. *Acta Psychiatrica scandinavica, suppl. 244.*

Slater, E. (1943) The neurotic constitution, a statistical study of two thousand neurotic soldiers. *Journal of Neurology and Psychiatry*, 6, 1–16.

Slater, E. (1947) Genetical causes of schizophrenic syndromes. *Monthly Review of Psychiatry and Neurology*, 113, 50–8.

Slater, E. (1950a) The genetic aspects of personality and neurosis. *Congrès international de psychiatrie à Paris 1950, Vol VI, Rapports.* Paris: Hermann, 119–54.

Slater, E. (1950b) Kriegserfahrungen und Psychopathiebegriff. *Monatsschrift für Psychiatrie und Neurologie*, 119, 207–26.

Slater, E. & Cowie, V. (1971) *The Genetics of Mental Disorders*. London, New York and Toronto: Oxford University Press.

Slater, E. and Glithero, E. (1965) A follow-up of patients diagnosed as suffering from 'hysteria'. *Journal of Psychosomatic Research*, 9, 9–13.

Slater, E. & Slater, P. (1944) A heuristic theory of neurosis. *Journal of Neurology and Psychiatry*, 7, 49–55.

Slater, E. & Tsuang, M. T. (1968) Abnormality on paternal and maternal sides: observations in Schizophrenia and manic-depression. *Journal of Medical Genetics*, 5, 197–9.

Stephens, D. A., Atkinson, M. W., Kay, D. W. K., Roth, M. & Garside, R. F. (1975) Psychiatric morbidity in parents and sibs of schizophrenics and non-schizophrenics. *British Journal of Psychiatry*, 127, 97–108.

Strömgren, E. (1968) Contributions to psychiatric epidemiology and genetics. *Acta jutlandica 40: 4, medical series*, 16.

Uddenberg, G. (1955) Diagnostic studies in prematures. Diss. Lund, and *Acta psychiatrica et neurlogica scandinavica, suppl. 104.*

Vanggaard, T. (1978) Diagnosis of schizophrenic borderline states. *Acta psychiatrica scandinavica*, 58, 213–30.

Wender, P. H. (1972) The minimal brain dysfunction syndrome in children. *Journal of Nervous and Mental Disease*, 155, 55–71.

A GENETIC BASIS FOR SOCIAL ATTITUDES?

H. J. Eysenck and Lindon Eaves

It used to be thought, in the words of W. S. Gilbert, that 'every boy and every girl that's born into this world alive is either a little Liberal or else a little Conservative'. Genetic theories like this one went out of favour after the First World War, and we have had, instead, theories stressing sociological and other environmental factors. Slowly the pendulum is swinging back, we hope to a balanced view that takes into account the interaction between genetic and environmental factors, a position long advocated by Eliot Slater. Surprising as it may seem, there is some evidence suggesting that social attitudes are influenced by genetic factors. Before discussing this evidence we will discuss social attitudes and their organization, and then suggest that this conclusion is not so unlikely as might be thought.

The study of social and political attitudes originated with the successful attempt of Thurstone to apply statistical methods to this field, and to work out inventories to measure them. Later work concentrated on the structure of social attitudes measured; it seemed likely that opinions about Jews, or negroes or women might not be independent of opinions about criminals, or permissiveness, or the death penalty. Indeed, common sense had long recognized there was a link; we talk readily about right and left in politics, or about conservatism and radicalism. These terms imply sets of correlated attitudes. Such hypotheses can be tested, and much work was done, both in America and England; to see whether such a generalization was tenable. The answer was both yes and no. Attitudes certainly cohere in recognizable and replicable patterns, but the hypothesis of one conservatism-liberalism factor was found to be over-simplified. There are at least three independent factors.

Two factors emerged prominently in *The Psychology of Politics* (Eysenck, 1954) where a number of statistical investigations were reported. Conservatism-radicalism, usually abbreviated to R for short, emerged as a powerful, broad-based factor; at the conservative end were religious attitudes, nationalist attitudes, ethnocentric and racist attitudes, and attitudes hostile to criminals and favouring stern treatment through birching and hanging. At the radical end were pacifist attitudes, attitudes favourable to world government, the giving up of national sovereignty, trial marriages, and sexual permissiveness. *The Psychology of Conservatism* (Wilson, 1973) has given strong support to the existence of a broad factor of this kind. We are dealing, though, with conservatism with a small 'c'. Working-class people emerge as more conservative than middle-class people, which at first sight seems strange because of the known support of the middle-class for the Conservative Party, and of the working-class for the Labour Party. But this support is related to Conservatism with a capital 'C', capitalist attitudes versus socialist attitudes. This socialism-capitalism factor later emerged as independent from conservatism. A person might hold conservative views on racialism, women in society, or permissiveness, and yet favour socialism and vote for the Labour Party, without logical contradiction. Indeed, on this socialism-capitalism factor working-class people favour socialism, middle-class people favour capitalism—including the economic measures associated with each. But we have nothing to say about this capitalist-socialist factor here, and we have only mentioned it to fill out the picture. A full discussion of the evidence for the distinction between conservatism and capitalism is given in Eysenck, 1971.

Another prominent factor (T), reported in *The Psychology of Politics* and in *The Psychology of Conservatism,* cut across the conservative-radical axis, and was labelled tender-mindedness versus tough-mindedness. It might also have been called liberalism versus authoritarianism, in line with the well-known 'authoritarian personality' concept, or idealism versus realism, the term preferred by Wilson. This T-Factor split the group of conservative and the group of radical attitudes in two. Tender-minded people held views favourable to idealistic, liberal causes—such as internationalism, religion, pacifism—while tough-minded people held attitudes of an authoritarian, manipulative kind, which might be regarded as more 'realistic'. Women and middle-class people were tender-minded; men and working-class people were tough-minded. Political parties were found to be grouped in the shape of a horseshoe—communists and fascists at the two ends, tough-minded radical and conservative respectively, with liberals at the tender-minded extreme, intermediate between right and left. Labour and Conservative party voters were left and right respectively on the R-axis and intermediate on the T-axis.

From the beginning it seemed likely that personality played an important part in tough-minded or tender-minded attitudes. The hypothesis was advanced and later verified that extraverts would be more tough-minded, introverts more tender-minded. Later work showed a connection between tough-mindedness and another personality factor, psychoticism (P). This connection was stronger than with extraversion (E). 'P' can be measured in non-pathological groups, and is characterized by hostile and aggressive behaviour, impersonal attitudes in interpersonal contact, coldness, and other behavioural indices (Eysenck and Eysenck, 1972). Psychotics and criminals, particularly those criminals convicted of crimes of violence, have been found to have exceptionally high P-scores, as do patients with behaviour disorders, and psychopaths (Eysenck and Eysenck, 1970; Verma and Eysenck, 1973). There is evidence that both E and P are genetically determined to a marked extent; several twin studies testify to this fact (Eysenck, 1974). If the relevant personality factors are genetically determined, and if personality determines social attitudes, then it is not so far-fetched to think that genes might be instrumental in determining social attitudes, at least as far as T is concerned.

Wilson had come to the conclusion that personality factors played an important part in the genesis of conservatism. He suggests that 'the conservative attitude syndrome serves an ego-defensive function, arising as a response to feelings of insecurity and inferiority, and a generalized fear of uncertainty (whether in terms of environmental complexity or the alternatives to action that are available)'. He postulates 'certain genetic factors', as well as certain environmental factors, as being responsible for a person's position on the conservatism-radicalism axis. These genetic factors cannot be identified with the personality measures we have used in our genetic studies.

Our study is simple to describe, but the analysis is complex. We administered two questionnaires to 451 pairs of monozygotic and 257 pairs of dizygotic same-sexed twins. One questionnaire contained measures of personality, in particular of neuroticism (N), extraversion (E), and psychoticism (P); the other contained measures of radicalism-conservatism, tender-mindedness versus tough mindedness, and a measure (Emphasis) of whether agreement or disagreement was strong or weak. We scored the questionnaires for the six factors and submitted the results to a joint statistical analysis, using adaptations of methods of biometrical genetical analysis pioneered by J. Jinks and other members of the Birmingham school of genetics (Mather and Jinks, 1971). These analyses are fully described in Eaves and Eysenck (1974) as are the assumptions made. We tested two hypotheses:

(1) All the observed trait variation and covariation can be attributed either to differences between the environmental influences shared by members of the same pair, or to differences in the environmental influences specific to individuals within the family. We called this the *simple environmental hypothesis*.

(2) All the variation and covariation can be attributed either to the cumulative and additive effects of many loci for which the population is polymorphic, or to specific environmental influences. We called this the *interactionist (genotype-environmental) hypothesis*.

The statistical tests showed that the simple environmental hypothesis failed to provide an adequate description of the variation and covariation of the six traits, P, E and N on the personality side and R, T and Emphasis. The interactionist model fitted the data reasonably well. The heritability estimates were as shown in Table 1.

These estimates are not corrected for unreliability of the measuring instrument which is added to the non-genetic variance. When the correction is made, the values given in the table are increased. We have not made the correction because the observed values establish the point that genetic factors are of importance in determining social attitudes, personality, and emphasis.

This analysis describes the variation of the six scores for each subject. Analysis of covariation tells us about the genetics of the interaction between the different scores. They confirm the correlation between extraversion and tough-mindedness, but add the stronger conclusion that the correlation has a genetical basis. Our findings show also that psychoticism is genetically and environmentally linked with tough-mindedness. Psychoticism is also associated with the Emphasis score; high scorers on P have a strong conviction of being right. Variability in this conviction is genetically determined to a significant degree. Radicalism, not unexpectedly, shows no significant covariation with any of the personality scores.

TABLE 1
Heritability estimates for social attitude and personality variables

	Heritability estimates
Radicalism	0·65
Tough-mindedness	0·54
Emphasis	0·37
Psychoticism	0·35
Extraversion	0·48
Neuroticism	0·49

Radicals tend to state their opinions more emphatically, a connection which also has a genetic basis.

Our study has some fairly straightforward findings. We found that a simple environmental hypothesis of the origin of social attitudes does not fit the facts. We found that genetic factors are important in determining the radical-conservatism and tender-mindedness versus tough-mindedness axes. We found that the strength with which a person holds his attitudes is in part genetical. We found that our personality factors are in large part determined genetically. And we found that there is a genetically caused inter-action between personality and social attitudes. High scorers on the E and P factors tend to be authoritarian and tough-minded. High scorers on P are predisposed to hold their attitudes with strength. Further work will be required to discover details of genetic mechanisms and to unearth the exact environmental factors relevant to the genesis of social attitudes. We doubt if such work will invalidate our conclusions.

References

Eaves, L. J. & Eysenck, H. J. (1974) Genetics and the development of social attitudes. *Nature,* **249,** 288-9.

Eysenck, H. J. (1954) *The Psychology of Politics.* London: Routledge and Kegan Paul.

Eysenck, H. J. (1972) *Psychology is about People.* London: Allen Lane, The Penguin Press.

Eysenck, H. J. (1975) The structure of social attitudes. *British Journal of Social and Clinical Psychology,* **14,** 323-31.

Eysenck, H. J. (1974) Genetic factors-personality development. In *Human Behaviour and Genetics* (ed A. R. Kaglan). Springfield: C. C. Thomas.

Eysenck, S. B. G. & Eysenck, H. J. (1970) Crime and personality: an empirical study of the three factor theory. *British Journal of Criminology,* **10,** 225-39.

Eysenck, S. B. G. & Eysenck, H. J. (1972) The questionnaire measurement of psychoticism. *Psychological Medicine,* **2,** 50-5.

Mather, K. & Jinks, J. L. (1971) *Biometrical Genetics.* London: Chapman and Hall.

Verma, R. M. & Eysenck, H. J. (1973) Severity and types of psychotic illness as a function of personality. *British Journal of Psychiatry,* **122,** 573-85.

Wilson, Glenn D. (1973) *The Psychology of Conservatism.* London: Academic Press.

THE GENETICS OF 3,000 CASES OF AFFECTIVE DISORDER

By P. Polonio

The history of the illness, the patient's previous adaptation, the present mental state and the outcome are the basis of diagnosis in psychiatry. A first attack of schizophrenia, for instance, may be mistaken for an affective disorder or thymopathy until the long-term outcome clarifies the true diagnosis. We have studied 3,000 patients with affective disorder diagnosed between 1930 and 1955. The median follow-up was 15 years, the last revision being in 1970. We report here observations on 2,824 of these cases and their families, from which we have made inferences about the genetical contribution to affective disorder.

We accept with reservations (Polonio, 1971) Kraepelin's initial description of manic-depressive insanity: 'the entire domain of periodic and circular insanity, simple mania, the greater part of morbid states termed melancholia, amentia and some minor or minimal mood swings (dysthymias), some periodic and some continuous. Dysthymias may be considered as the rudiments of more severe disease and they merge without a clear boundary into normal variations of mood'. Kraepelin described all these polymorphic states as variations in the expression of a single morbid process, but accepted that subordinate groups might be isolated eventually. Even if this happened, all the symptoms he described would continue to belong to the clinical picture of 'manic-depressive insanity', an illness he believed to be mainly constitutional or genetical, discounting the importance of psychological causality. 'Manic-depressive insanity may be to an astonishing degree independent of external influences.'

The duration of the illnesses in our sample varied from one week, when death occurred in the first attack, to 63 years, summing overall to 42,060 years which includes illness-free intervals. My co-workers and I attempted to classify our material diagnostically, and by intensity of symptoms, dominant symptoms, age of onset, number of attacks and their duration. Each patient was studied by one of my collaborators and by me as to diagnosis and classification. Our sample comprised inpatients and corresponded fairly well to Kraepelin's description.

Results
A first attack had a bimodal distribution, the first peak being at 20–24 years, the second at 40–44. Many women and some men began their illnesses at the time of the climacteric and were classified as involutional depression. These observations, as well as many other characteristics of our sample, accord with the usual distribution of manic-depressive insanity and enable us to consider it as representative, even though outpatients have been excluded.

Diagnosis, given adequate follow-up, is a simple matter, but other aims are difficult to achieve. In the end, we used two groups, one of good and one of poor prognosis. We distinguished a nuclear group of 1,820 cases comprising 20 per cent depressions, 15 per cent periodic depressions, 13 per cent mania, 6 per cent periodic mania and 46 per cent cyclothymia. We classified the remaining 1,004 patients into three subgroups: the first comprising involutional depression 4 per cent, anxiety depression 32 per cent, hypochondriacal depression 6 per cent, and obsessive depression 9 per cent. The second subgroup was small and included chronic depression 4 per cent, chronic mania 2 per cent, delusional and confusional thymopathy 1 per cent. the third subgroup was made up of atypical depression 9 per cent, atypical mania 2 per cent, and reactive depression 11 per cent.

The nuclear group had the highest incidence of a history of familial thymopathy: 74 per cent among cases of periodic mania, 64 per cent of cases of cyclothymia, and 61 per cent of cases with periodic depression. Outside this nuclear group the incidence of thymopathy in the family was lower (43 per cent), except obsessive thymopathy (71 per cent of the 89 cases).

Involutional depression had a familial incidence of thymopathic disorder of 48 per cent, anxiety depression 45 per cent, and hypochondriacal depression 34 per cent. These percentages are statistically lower than the percentages observed in the nuclear group. The importance of genetic predisposition in symptomatic and reactive depressions is demonstrated by our finding that in 53 symptomatic depressions the incidence of thymopathy in the family was 60 per cent, and in the 113 reactive depressions 58 per cent. In the remaining 390 cases the incidence of family thymopathy was 35 per cent. These 390 cases comprised the so-called polymorphic depressions of Kraepelin, pseudo-neurotic depressions, masked depressions, smiling depressions and psychosomatic depressions, all of which had a lower incidence of a history of thymopathy in the family.

Taken together, the findings of these various groups suggest the existence of a continuum of thymopathies determined by genetical factors of a quantitatively graded kind.

By and large, prognosis was unrelated to the existence of thymopathy in the family, excepting nuclear cases. The prognosis here was twice as bad in those with such a history as in those who did not have a family history of thymopathy. We tried to individualize Weitbrecht endo-reactive depressions, but structural analysis and follow-up led us to include them with simple depressions, together with the many reactive and symptomatic disorders.

We were unable to compare unipolar with bipolar thymopathy. The reason is this: many so-called unipolar manic or depressive disorders show an occasional swing in the opposing direction, especially late in life. Moreover, patients may be diagnosed periodic mania and depression according to the dominant mood swing, since patients who need to be hospitalized only during the manic or depressive phase may be so labelled only because the opposite swing which occurred was well tolerated by the patient and those in his immediate environment. Further, some patients were considered as depressions even though occasional manic attacks were recorded.

As to the possible existence of unipolar thymopathy, we distinguished three groups of such mood disturbances in our studies. But it must be recalled that 40 years or more may elapse before a typical periodic depression develops manic attacks which change the diagnosis from periodic depression to cyclothymia. We were not, therefore, able to reach any conclusion.

We found 60 patients among the direct descendants of 160 thymopathic men. Fifty-two per cent were males and their illnesses were twice as severe as that for the group as a whole. Among the direct descendants of 452 thymopathic women there were 119 patients, but their prognosis did not depart from the overall. We believe this indicates a sex-linked influence, as has already been suggested by Rüdin (unpublished material), and by Winokur and Reich (1969) as well as many others.

Affective disorders are not to be explained by one exclusive cause. There are probably several genetic disturbances that lead to thymopathy, and somatic and psychological causes as well. For example, we have seen typical thymopathic syndromes among patients who have epilepsy, which may respond well to antidepressant treatment. Reactive depressions which, it may be recalled, have a marked family history of thymopathic disorder may also respond well to antidepressant treatment.

We turn now to discuss other mental illnesses found among the families of our sample of affective disorders. Schizophrenia was present in 2 per cent of the families, epilepsy in 2.6 per cent. Alcoholism reached 10 per cent as compared to 3 per cent in the general population. However, it is difficult to evaluate such a finding, since alcohol abuse is widespread in Portugal. Anyone who drinks too much and has a psychiatric illness in the family is considered alcoholic. Heavy drinking, it should be remembered, is a way of alleviating symptoms in thymopathy and chronic alcoholism may come to seem to be the principal disease, a substitute illness for thymopathy.

In 4 per cent of the families of the whole sample we found chronic psychosis and dementia. Such a family history seemed unrelated to the prognosis, but the number is too small to allow confident conclusions to be drawn. Besides, our knowledge of familial cases was incomplete. In such chronic patients affective disorder could be a reaction of the organism in Bonhoeffer's sense: a reaction which could explain too the frequent depressive states found in late schizophrenia (Polonio, 1954).

Discussion

It is possible, as Kraepelin said in his clinical description, to try and explain all our findings by a single cause. But we accept, as he accepted, that there are several thymopathic diseases, besides affective syndromes and reactions. Any trigger, as described by Bonhoeffer, may set in motion such reactions. The duration of the event and its more or less massive effect influences the course of the reaction.

The general description of manic-depressive psychosis, considered by the English-speaking countries as affective disorder, still stands up to the test of history taking and follow-up. Kraepelin accepted the possibility of the existence of several subgroups, but manic-depressive insanity as a clinical entity still exists as he described it.

A pathological mood disorder due to many causes that we cannot yet identify seems possible in all men. The terms 'schizophrenia' and 'manic-depressive psychosis' must encompass clinical entities with specific aetiologies, and syndromes and reactions of a diverse causation, but as yet we have no classification based on aetiology. In 50 per cent of families of our patients we found evidence of thymopathic disease, and if we consider only nuclear cases this proportion reaches 61 per cent, increasing to 75 per cent in cases of periodic mania, which, although suggesting a dominant transmission, still allows of other possibilities (Slater, 1938).

We have freely used the terms thymopathy, thymopathic and

thymic diseases. They have the same meaning as affective or mood disorder, but are more precise and correspond more closely to our understanding of these illnesses than do the terms manic-depressive psychosis or manic-depressive insanity. Besides, these last two terms sound unsatisfactory and untrue to both patient and his doctor. Patients prefer to hear they have a thymopathy rather than a manic-depressive psychosis.

Summary

Our findings suggest there are three kinds of genetically determined thymopathy: dominant, sex-linked and polygenic. As reactions, thymopathies can be seen in symptomatic psychosis, schizophrenia and epilepsy, which indicates that other factors than a genetic cause must be important.

Acknowledgements

My co-workers were the late M. Figueiredo, the late P. Silva, F. Mendes, L. Eglesias, A. Galvão and A. Ribeiro. The statistical study was made by P. Mello and J. Polonio. The social services of the Julio de Matos Hospital and the Institute of Mental Health under the guidance of M. G. Salles assisted us with our studies.

References

Polonio, P. (1954) Involutional schizophrenia. *Diseases of the Nervous System*, XV, 10–11.

Polonio, P. (1971) Body–mind problems from an empirical point of view. *British Journal of Psychiatry*, 118, 7–10.

Slater, E. (1938) Zur Erbpathologie des manisch depressive Irresein. *Zeitschrift für Neurologie und Psychiatrie*, 163, 1–47.

Winokur, G. & Tanna, V. L. (1969) Possible role of X-linked dominant factor. *Diseases of the Nervous System*, 30/2, 89–94.

PATHOGRAPHY

EDVARD MUNCH

A PSYCHIATRIC OUTLINE

Einar Kringlen

In Edvard Munch, Norway's greatest painter, life and art were inseparable. Munch painted what he felt, and much of his work reflects his gloomy childhood years and the conflicts which he struggled with all his life.

What was Munch like as a person? Of all the great Western painters Munch is perhaps the least known with regard to the relation between his life and his art. Compared with van Gogh and Gauguin, for instance, there is not much written about him. But it is difficult to arrive at an accurate perception of him because he kept people at a distance. Rolf Stenersen has provided an intimate biography of Munch's later years, since he knew the artist during the last twenty years of his life. Strangely, there are no descriptions of a more detailed character of Munch as a young or middle-aged man, and Stenersen is not reliable here.

Some biographical notes
Edvard Munch was born in 1863 and died in 1944 aged eighty. On the paternal side he was descended from an intellectual family. His father, a brother of the great historian, P. A. Munch, practised medicine in the slum area of Oslo. Because he frequently refused to receive money for his work the family had a modest income and the children were expected to live frugally.

Edvard was the second of five children. From an early age he was well acquainted with misery, disease and death. When he was five, his mother died of tuberculosis. He was often ill with bronchitis which frequently kept him in bed with fever. Now and then Edvard would accompany his father on visits to patients in their homes. When he was thirteen, his elder sister Sophie died, also of tuberculosis. Another sister, Laura, suffered from periodic depression and died in a mental institution. His only brother Andreas died of tuberculosis as a young man. Munch's relationship with his remaining sister Inger was always harmonious.

His mother's sister took over the household after his mother died. The aunt was a good support for Edvard and she encouraged his artistic spirit. Nevertheless, Edvard always felt that his childhood had been bleak and miserable, that he had been treated unjustly, first of all by the loss of his mother, and then by having a father who was so strict.

The father, by nature a religious man who always had a serious attitude to life, became dejected after his wife's death. He brooded over sin and eternal punishment, frequently threatening the children with the torments of hell if they did not follow the strait and narrow path. There is no indication that he was treated for a manic-depressive psychosis; however, from a clinical point of view his behaviour seems to fit the diagnosis. He wandered around for long periods pacing the floor in anxious despair, melancholic and downcast. When he felt he had to punish his children, he could develop fits or paroxysms of rage.

At the age of seventeen Edvard enrolled in the Technical School of Oslo on his father's advice. The father would have wanted him to study at the University, but because of his skill at drawing it was thought he would make a good engineer. However, because of his spells of bronchitis, Edvard was unable to attend the School regularly, and because his interests turned more and more to painting, his father allowed him to leave school in the first year. His aunt Laura was instrumental in this development.

Together with some friends, Edvard rented a studio in Oslo. Some of his best-known pictures, for instance 'Sick Girl', were painted in this early period. Christiania, as Oslo was then called, was a provincial town with less than 100,000 inhabitants. So in 1885, when 22, he went to Paris for a few weeks. Four years later he returned there, particularly to study the old masters, Goya Rembrandt and Velasquez. He was also most impressed by what he saw of van Gogh's work.

When Munch was 27, his father died. Munch's relationship with his father was at times strained, but he never broke with him and the bereavement was a hard blow and came to influence his philosophy of life and artistic development. His literary notes from this period are numerous, and one can observe how after the death of his father Munch re-experiences his difficult childhood and gradually distances the conflicts. Simultaneously Munch broke away from naturalism. He wrote: 'No longer should one paint interiors, people who read, women who knit, instead one should paint living individuals who breathe and feel, suffer and love'.

In 1892, at the age of 29, Munch was invited to Berlin to exhibit. His exhibition became a scandal and was closed. The conservative elements of the Art Society thought his paintings were too shocking. Despite his hardships in Berlin, he enjoyed the city and stayed three years, but briefly visited Copenhagen, Dresden, Munich and Stockholm.

The years 1899-1905 are characterized by Munch's restless travelling in Europe, with shorter stays in Norway during the summer. He moved from hotel to hotel, lived an irregular life, drank and smoked heavily, but at the same time worked extremely hard, exhibiting in Norway, Germany, France, Italy, Switzerland, and even in the United States of America. From 1892 to 1905 he had more than a hundred exhibitions in Europe and North America (Hodin, 1972).

From 1902 until 1908 Munch was severely mentally disturbed, unbalanced and suspicious, which led to his being involved in a series of brawls. Once, for instance, he nearly killed an artist friend. Several times he received treatment in German sanatoria. In 1908 he was admitted to Dr Jacobsen's clinic in Copenhagen and stayed eight months. After 1908, he settled down in Norway, bought a summer house in the southern part of the country, and started, so to speak, a new life. It would appear that his style of painting also changed. His pictures became more colourful, focusing more attention on form than content. Ragna Stang (1977) maintains that Munch's painting style had changed before 1908.* His working capacity seemed to be in top gear during these years. He received a series of assignments and finished the Aula pictures for the University of Oslo.

By 1930, now approaching 70, he was troubled by an eye disease which returned eight years later and almost blinded him. During these eight years he seems to have been nervous, restless and anxious. He died, when a common cold developed into bronchitis and pneumonia on January 23, 1944.

What was Munch like as a person?
Munch was unusually handsome, the kind of man one turns around to look at in the street: tall, slim, with a distinctive and sensitive face. His older colleague, Christian Krogh, called him 'pretty Edvard', but also 'stupid Edvard'. Munch indeed had in his makeup, as had so many great artists and scientists, a mixture of scepticism and credulity.

*Many who have written about Munch from a psychiatric point of view have been unaware of the fact that Munch's style had changed before his breakdown in 1908. See Huggler (1958) and Steinberg and Weiss (1954).

People who have known Munch and written about him have described him as a shy and seclusive man, more of an observer than a participant. In the company of friends, he was taciturn and observed what was going on, but seldom said much, except for ironical utterances against himself. Because he kept people at a distance, he was thought to be arrogant. It was also typical of him that he reacted strongly, with haughty contempt, to any criticism he felt unjust.

In a personal encounter with a model, a visitor or a friend he talked a lot to avoid critical remarks or attacks. To his friend, the anatomist Professor Schreiner (1946) he said: 'I talk very much as all nervous people do; when speaking I imprison the person and hinder his attack on me . . . I use speech as a defensive weapon'.

Relationship with men
Munch's relationship with men was strained. He actually hated his mentor, the somewhat older painter, Christian Krogh, a hatred which certainly had an irrational basis. Perhaps he perceived Christian Krogh as a sort of father figure. On the other hand he was a god-parent to Krogh's son. In general, Edvard Munch stayed away from painters in Norway and kept company with literary men. However, Munch enjoyed the friendship of several painters on the continent, particularly in Germany. The only Norwegian painter he cultivated was Ludwig Karsten whom he once nearly killed by shooting at him. He seemed to enjoy the company of the Norwegian poet Sigbjörn Obstfelder, a schizoid, sensitive man who often would sit with Munch, watching him paint, without saying anything. Obstfelder later on developed a schizophrenic psychosis.

Munch's friendship with the writer Jappe Nilsen must be mentioned, because this friendship endured many crises and lasted more than forty years. Munch was 25 when he met the 17-year-old Jappe Nilsen. During the many restless years when Munch roamed the continent, he never lost contact with him. While a patient in Dr Jacobsen's clinic, Munch received several letters from Nilsen who acted as the best kind of supportive therapist, listening to Munch's paranoid accusations but never accepting them. Instead he tried to explain to Munch how and why he was wrong. Munch maintained, for instance, that there had been a plot against him. Jappe Nilsen pointed out that Munch himself had been provocative toward his friends, and that the various incidents he mentioned were not expressions of a massive, systematic plot, but coincidences. 'There was never a plot against you', Nilsen assured his friend in a letter.

Munch's relationship with Strindberg was odd and not without comical aspects. Both had paranoid tendencies. Munch adored Strindberg and considered him a genius. Although they were good friends, they were, at times, afraid of each other. In his 'Inferno' period in Paris, Strindberg thought that Munch would asphyxiate him with poisonous gas. And Munch, one day when he and Strindberg were eating at a sidewalk café together, suddenly shook off his coat (he had borrowed it from Strindberg) and left the café. He had all at once begun to feel uncomfortable and trembly in his friend's overcoat, and apparently ascribed his bodily sensations to Strindberg's personality (Burnham, 1973).

Relationship with women

If Munch's relationship with men was fraught with conflict, so too was his relationship with women. Women found him very attractive and some tried to win him. But he always managed to escape and remained a bachelor all his life. Very little is known about his intimate life with women. We do know that he was rather reserved even with women whom he knew fairly well. He had several love affairs as we shall see, but it was his habit to break them off abruptly.

Munch visited brothels, as did other artists of the time, but he seemed to feel panic whenever his relationship with a woman threatened to become too close.

Munch's motivation not to marry was probably determined by many factors. He believed he was descended from a genetically sick family, a belief reinforced by medical opinion. However, more important were his fears of emotional binding to another person and of marriage threatening his artistic creativity. Love was for Munch combined with pain; he even compared love with death (Burkhardt, 1965).

> It was as if each time a woman showed him tenderness he was reminded of his mother who at her deathbed had smiled at him and stroked his hair. According to Stenersen this image of the dying mother seemed to interfere with any intimate contact with other women. Perhaps also his incestuous longing for his younger sister interfered with his relationship with other women. One of his pictures of his sister Inger shows a beautiful sensual young woman. Munch was reluctant to sign this picture. When discussing the matter with Stenersen he admitted his strong urge to kiss the well-rounded lips.
>
> Munch seems as a young man to have been in love with his aunt Laura who came to care for the family after the mother died. Once, having painted her with a white dot in her ear, Munch asked Stenersen: 'Do you know what this is?' 'A white dot.' 'No, it is a kiss.' Munch painted his aunt as being much younger than she actually was. Yet, despite all she had done for him, he in later years expressed the feeling that she had failed him. Most likely Munch's father did not marry Laura, which would have been sensible, because he realized that his son was fond of her.

According to his diaries. Munch fell in love with a married woman when he was 22, obviously a significant experience for the young artist. Munch had several rendezvous with this woman in the forest (note his many paintings of women and trees) but there is evidence that he identified with her husband, and in a way this love affair reinforced his view of women as faithless and treacherous creatures.

The picture 'Lady with a Brooch' is one of Munch's most captivating pictures, evidently painted by a man in love. The woman is Eva Mudoci, a British violinist whom Jappe Nilsen suggested Munch should court to save her from her relationship with the American pianist Bela Edwards. Munch yielded to his friend's advice, and succeeded in getting Eva Mudoci to fall in love with him. Thus the idea which had started as a jest became serious. Most likely the feelings of sympathy and love were reciprocal, and an intimate relationship developed. But then while they were travelling together from Oslo to Copenhagen, Munch suddenly left the train without his baggage. Eva Mudoci had touched on the question of marriage, and this possibility apparently frightened the artist. Munch was not able to tolerate a binding relationship which for him meant that he could be 'devoured' or later on abandoned. 'Unhappiness and misery follows the woman,' as he noted in his diary. 'To stay away from her is the best.' His mother had abandoned him when he was five. His older sister had left him when he was thirteen. His friend Jappe Nilsen had experienced love, but had been betrayed and left with a broken heart. And had not his brother, Andreas, died young, just after he had been married for six months? Woman was a dangerous creature that one should stay away from. His brother had been 'too weak for marriage'. It was the woman who had wanted marriage. Munch had too often experienced the loss of those whom he loved most. Moreover he had fantasies about women—for instance, that they wanted the whole man. A man's work could suffer from such a relationship. Sexual intercourse was similar to intercourse with death. A man associating with a woman kills something within himself. Several paintings reveal this theme.

From 1898 to 1902, when he was 39, Munch was in love with Tulla Larsen, a merchant's daughter in Christiania; but he was afraid of tying himself to the girl forever, and tried to separate from her. She was desperately in love with Munch and tried in every way to maintain his interest. Once his friends arranged a macabre performance. The woman was put on her deathbed and Munch was sent for, the message being that she was dying. When Munch arrived, she suddenly stood up, whereupon he turned away from her in rage, deeply hurt. However, she accompanied him back to his house, where she tried to shoot herself. But Munch managed to grab the pistol, in the process having part of one of his left fingers shot off.

After this episode, Munch's attitude toward women became bitter and irreconcilable.

Neurosis and paranoid psychosis

Munch was an eccentric in a number of ways. He would sometimes put his paintings on the floor and then walk over them. He frequently hung them outdoors in cold and rainy weather—the 'horse cure'—as he called it. He seemed to have been suspicious, with a tendency to self-reference, from youth onward. He considered himself nervous and weak. He had inherited his nervousness from his father, and his bad lungs from his mother, he said. He had a terror of the dark and suffered from agoraphobia. He would, for instance, walk close to walls and had difficulty in crossing a street without alcoholic fortification. Particularly during his middle years, he was afflicted with 'heart trouble' and fits of dizziness. All his life he was troubled by sleeplessness. He might suddenly buy a ticket for the sleeper to Stockholm from Oslo because he knew that he slept well on the train.

Munch seemed intuitively to realize that his artistic creativity was based upon his neurotic conflicts. His friend, the anatomist Schreiner, would very much have liked to help him, but Munch was ambivalent about being 'cured', afraid of losing his artistic gift if he gave up his mental problems. Through his painting he was able to abreact his emotional conflicts. Painting was a sort of psychotherapy through which he was able to gain emotional balance. Munch often mentions how nervousness accompanied him through life. When he painted 'The Shriek' he instinctly used his fear in order to free himself from anxiety. Munch felt that his mental problems were necessity for him. 'Without anxiety and disease I would have been as a ship without a helm.'

During his restless wandering years on the continent he worked hard. He drank heavily during these years, at night to get sleepy, and in the morning to get awake, as he said. But, clinically speaking, he was hardly an alcoholic. There are no reports of delirium tremens, no information concerning damage to his liver and, more significantly, he abstained from alcohol for many years after his stay in Dr Jacobsen's clinic. He lived to be eighty which would have been unusual if he were an alcoholic.

Was Munch schizophrenic? Not in the strict clinical sense of the word. He was by nature paranoid and his behaviour was often psychotic, but he was always able to pull himself together again. There was no sign of the usual deteriorating autistic thinking and extreme withdrawal from other people. When he was admitted to Dr Jacobsen's clinic on December 1, 1908, he was clearly psychotic. He had for several years been troubled with exaggerated ideas of reference. He felt people were talking behind his back, that this or that person spread lies about him. And he sometimes thought that people believed him to be homosexual. He would sit in a café and suddenly rise from his seat, cross over to another table and strike a person because he felt that person was talking about him. At times he felt he was being followed and persecuted. Because of his paranoid attitude he frequently got into fights with other painters. Before he was admitted to Jacobsen's clinic, he thought that Jacobsen was the centre of a plot against him. Jappe Nilsen tried to correct him, pointing out that he had always been the provoking agent. In one fight, he told Munch that he had insulted, mocked and ridiculed a man, before being struck in retaliation.

Munch's breakdown in 1908 might be considered a reactive paranoid psychosis, precipitated by a series of stresses, such as heavy drinking, social isolation, and stormy love affairs. It represented the culmination of a crisis which had lasted for many years. He could never forget the woman who had shot off part of his finger and talked about it to his friends constantly. One must also bear in mind that he had been under constant attack from the bourgeois press and conservative critics since he was 23, his art being described as pathological and the work of a madman. Even the well-known Norwegian psychiatrist Johan Scharffenberg had said so. The direct precipitant of his mental breakdown was a wild drinking bout which he had with a friend.

Munch stayed eight months at the clinic in Copenhagen, receiving physical treatment and free of responsibilities. Nevertheless he worked as never before at his paintings. In the summer of 1909, when 46, he returned to Norway, restored and full of initiative, but at the same time fearful and on his guard. He bought a house on the southern coast of Norway and started a new life. He always considered the Copenhagen period the end of a phase in his life.

Munch never became free of psychic troubles. Throughout his life his hypersensitive personality and paranoid attitude created interpersonal problems. He kept neighbours and colleagues at a distance and often behaved strangely. As he approached old age he often expressed a sadness at being old, and a fear of death. During his last years he was nervous, suspicious and difficult.

When he died, he left over 2,000 paintings, 5,000 drawings and sketches, and more than 50,000 prints, a remarkable production.

We do not know enough to give a satisfactory explanation of what led to Munch's extreme hypersensitivity, and of how this in turn led to a paranoid psychosis; but we can point to several life circumstances which are usually connected with mental illness in general— a dismal childhood, loss of his mother, a strict upbringing, conflicts with his father (which may have sensitized him to later criticism in the press) and complications in his formative human relationships. Early relationships with significant people, parents, sisters or brothers, determine to a large degree relationships with people in adult life. I have indicated how Munch's relations with his mother and sisters may have made it difficult for him as a man to relate intimately with women, and I have suggested how his relationship with his father came to shape his relations with other men.

'No paranoid psychosis unless there is guilt feeling', it has been said. In Munch's case it is easy to see how circumstances must have created guilt feelings. His bohemian life, his association with deviant artists, alcoholics and prostitutes sharply contrasted with the values he had been taught as a boy. He knew that his life style was in opposition to all his father's wishes. This new manner of living must have created conflicts and identity problems in the young man. Later on the criticism of his art by influential newspapers must have reinforced his uncertainty and further shaken his self-esteem.

Hypersensitivity and uncertainty are just those personality traits that dispose to paranoid psychosis. Many events in Munch's life are typical precipitating factors in the development of paranoid psychosis, events which would engender uncertainty, particularly within the sexual sphere, and those which isolate the individual from his group. He also abused himself physically, lived an irregular life, worked too hard and drank too much. All this must have affected his mental state.

Ideas of reference are often elicited in sensitive individuals by moral failures which in turn produce guilt and expectations of punishment. The gap between this state and a paranoid system is not wide.

The content of a paranoid psychosis reflects the individual's problems. Freud maintained that paranoid ideas were due to latent homosexual impulses, a theory that today is not accepted by many clinicians. Generally, the content of the paranoid ideas will be determined by the type of conflicts the individual suffers. Homosexual thoughts may dominate if the patient's identity confusion expresses itself in doubt with regard to his own sexual identity. In Munch's case the paranoid ideas were of a varied nature—sometimes people were plotting against him, at other times they were whispering, lying and talking negatively about him, and even maintaining that he was homosexual. There are, however, no indications that Munch had any homosexual relationships.

I have attempted to give a picture of the person Edvard Munch. I have not touched on the quality of his art, nor have I discussed in depth his art in relation to his mental functioning. Many have found his earlier pictures macabre. However, these works reveal better than words his emotional conflicts, his fear of death, his identity conflicts, his feeling of loneliness and isolation, his fear of closeness, his jealousy. Munch's fear of death is revealed in many ways. He did not like sunsets. 'I get cold when I observe the sun's fall. Everything gets quiet. I do not like to witness something die'. His sadness is shown in his seascapes, where the moon is central and the violet colour reinforces the impression of melancholy and *tristesse*. The arrangement of elements in the pictures expresses loneliness and separation, even to the extent of people turning away from each other.

Life and art represented opposing poles in Munch's psyche. As Ragna Stang (1977) points out, in Munch's restless and relatively extraverted period his art had an introverted and expressive quality, whereas, later on, when his artistic development took on a more extraverted direction, Munch withdrew from the external world.

Many of Munch's paintings have an extreme emotional intensity. The people in his pictures express anguish, desperation and loneliness, so do the landscape, the sea, the forest, the sky. It was Munch's sensitivity to all he beheld that enabled him to achieve this intensity.

References

Burkhardt, H. (1965) Angst und Eros bei Edvard Munch. *Deutsch. Ärztbl.,* **62,** 2098–2102.

Burnham, D. L. (1973) Strindberg's 'Inferno' and Sullivan's 'extravasation of meaning'. *Cont. Psychoan.,* **9,** 190–208.

Hodin, J. P. (1972) *Edvard Munch.* London.

Huggler, M. (1958) Die Überwindung der Lebensangst im Werk von Edvard Munch. *Conf. Psychiat.,* **1,** 3–16.

Schreiner, K. E. (1946) Minner fra Ekely. In: *Edvard Munch som vi kjente ham.* Oslo: Dreyer.

Stang, R. (1977) *Edvard Munch. Mennesket og kunstneren.* Oslo: Aschehoug. (English edition (1979) London: Frazer.)

Steinberg, S. & Weiss, J. (1954). The art of Edvard Munch and its function in his mental life. *Psychoan. Quart,* **23,** 409–423.

Strindberg, A. (1897) *Inferno.* London: Hutchinson (1962).

'THE PSYCHOPATHOLOGY OF A CORRESPONDENCE COLUMN'

Denis Leigh

It is all too easy to identify a man with his major contribution to his subject, and to forget those aspects of his work which seem to be of marginal significance. Eliot Slater, for many, is identified with his work on genetics—but to those of us who have known him for a quarter of a century it is the many-sided nature of the man which is of major interest. In 1947 an intriguing paper appeared in the *British Journal of Medical Psychology* entitled 'The psychopathology of a correspondence column', co-authored by Eliot Slater and a hand-writing expert, M. J. Mannheim. In those days there was some interest in handwriting and its relationship to personality and psychiatric disorder. Erich Guttman had presented me in 1946 with a copy of *Handschrift und Karacter* by Ludwig Klages, and specimens of our patients' handwriting were often included in the clinical notes. As for sexual deviation—that was a specialized and perhaps somewhat disreputable and anecdotal field of psychiatry to be interested in—at least that was the impression I had gained in my first two years at the Maudsley. Characteristically Eliot Slater had had the knowledge and the intellectual curiosity to seize upon a curious correspondence which had been published in a contemporary popular illustrated weekly. It was concerned with corporal punishment; and had begun with a letter from a lady complaining of the habits of modern girls (the 1939 version), in particular of the fashion for wearing shorts. They needed a good caning, she wrote. There had been such an immediate and over-whelming flood of letters in response, that the correspondence had had to be closed by the editor after four weeks. The journal had never received a larger number of letters on any subject. Slater was intrigued, obtained the letters and set to work: 347 letters from 432 separate individuals were analysed. The paper itself must be read in detail; suffice it to say that using statistical methods and graphological analysis, it was concluded that sadism and masochism were to be regarded as distinct qualities, arising in personalities of very different structure. As a contribution to the literature on sado-masochism, the paper was perhaps the first to employ any kind of objective approach to the subject.

For many years I had been intrigued by the character and career of T. E. Lawrence. I had visited Syria, the Lebanon and Jordan, seen the rusting rails and dilapidated culverts of the Trans-Hejaz Railway, explored Maan, the scene of one of his pitched battles against the Turks, and ridden into Petra. The road to Akaba stretched into the desert before me—it was not hard to visualize El-Aurens entering Damascus where there were tanks in the streets at the time of my visit. In 1968 a unique opportunity arose to make a closer study of this remarkable man. The *Sunday Times* had mounted a careful investigation of certain aspects of Lawrence's life following an approach to the paper by Mr John Bruce, who claimed to have known Lawrence since 1922, and to have been involved in an extraordinary relationship with him. Informants had been sought and questioned; the family of the Bey of Deraa, he who had supposedly inflicted such a serious mental trauma on Lawrence, had been contacted, the Bey's diaries had been read, old soldiers and comrades had been traced and interviewed; and new documentary evidence had been consulted. The mass of written information already available on Lawrence was now supplemented by material based on reasonably objective information. It had become possible to attempt to piece together Colonel Lawrence's medical and psychiatric history, based on contemporary records and on the accounts of his personal acquaintances.

Previously it had been alleged that Lawrence had been a pathological liar and braggart; that he had been a homosexual, an exhibitionist and a fraud. That as a result of a sadistically homosexual assault at Deraa his whole mental life had been transformed and he had become a broken man. According to Mr Bruce, Lawrence had involved him in a curiously complex situation. Lawrence told him that he (Lawrence) was to be punished by the 'Old Man'—some sort of distant relative whose displeasure Lawrence had aroused. As part of the punishment Lawrence was to be flogged by Bruce. Between 1923 and 1935 there were nine flogging episodes, with Bruce using a birch, at first applied over the trousers but later on the bare buttocks. Bruce was 19 when he met the nearly 34-year-old Lawrence and the relationship lasted nearly 13 years. It was curiously reminiscent of an earlier happier relation with Dahoum, a Syrian donkey-boy, whom Lawrence had met whilst excavating at Carchemish in 1911, and whom he had brought back with him to England. Dahoum had been recruited by Lawrence as an agent, trained as a photographer, and had almost certainly died in Lawrence's service in 1918. It had been to Salim Ahmed, alias Dahoum, that *Seven Pillars* is believed to have been dedicated. Was it possible that in the relationship with Bruce, Lawrence was recreating this earlier situation—but now with overtones of guilt and remorse resulting from Dahoum's death, and demanding punishment and expiation? It is a simplification to regard masochistic activity as predominantly sexual in nature. Particularly in such a complex man as Lawrence, the masochistic rituals may contain elements of moral masochism, of self-degradation, and of mourning—as well as exerting a therapeutic effect in the relief of tension, or the relief of too much suffering. Slater had pointed out that the analysis of the graphological characteristics of the letters in his correspondence showed that the masochistic character differed from the sadistic. The masochistic character was 'more subject to anxiety conditions, worry and moodiness, and to self-centredness and isolation', whilst the sadistic was more mature than the average, much more aggressive, colder and more egotistical and more frequently showed a tendency to instability, lack of self-control and moral weakness. His findings did not support the generally accepted view that sadism and masochism were polar qualities frequently shown in the same individual. In fact Mannheim and Slater were led to the opposite conclusions, that sadism and masochism were independent tendencies, not particularly frequently associated together. Certainly in Lawrence there never were any indications of sadism— the massacre on the Turkish force at Tafas had been held to sully his honour; but in the heat of battle, what is a soldier's duty but to win and kill? And that cannot be regarded as sadistic.

There is another aspect to Lawrence's life which must be taken into account when considering this problem of his beatings. He was worn out, physically and mentally at the end of the war. He was down to under six stone in weight, he had lost two brothers in action, and six months after he left Damascus his father had died in the great influenza epidemic. He yet had to endure the struggle on behalf of the Arab cause at the Peace Conference, to write *Seven Pillars* and to see his hopes dashed to the ground—Feisal thrown out of Syria by the French and the old King Hussein defeated by Ibn Saud and exiled to Cyprus. Despite everything he struggled on for a further five years, before finding that extraordinary solution to his problems, enlistment in the ranks of the Royal Air Force. I have suggested that the clinical picture at this time was that of a man suffering from a depressive illness in which guilt and self-reproach were prominent features. The punishment he arranged for himself, so similar to some of the primitive treatments for depression employed over the centuries, may have had a therapeutic effect. So many of our patients in their depression long for a release from responsibility, from the bonds of their ordinary daily existence; at the same time unable unequivocally to give up a life pattern which has given them much satisfaction. So it was with Lawrence—sinking to the bottom, seeking anonymity in the ranks, yet maintaining his relationships with the men of power and of the pen, ambivalent about his former exploits.

This type of study—the pathography of a genius, is to-day relatively uncommon in the psychiatric literature, other than the psychoanalytical. Again Eliot Slater has brought his special qualities to bear on the life of Robert Schumann. With Alfred Meyer (1959) he analysed and charted Schumann's musical productivity—linking it with the chronology of his known mood changes; Schumann's first illness was also analysed and diagnosed. The application of scientific methods to the study of human nature has been one of the characteristics of the Maudsley School of Psychiatry. Slater has shown that such methods can be applied to pathography and to certain behavioural traits such as sadism and masochism. In my own studies of T. E. Lawrence the example of Eliot Slater has been a strong influence in the avoidance of speculation and of psychodynamic constructions based on fragmentary information. In his next decade perhaps he will consider a graphological and content analysis of some of Lawrence's letters.

References

Knightley, P. & Simpson, C. (1969) *The Secret Lives of Lawrence of Arabia*. London: Nelson.

Mannheim, M. J. & Slater, Eliot (1947) The Psychopathology of a Correspondence Column. *Brit. J. Med. Psych.,* **xxi,** 50.

Slater, Eliot & Meyer, Alfred (1959) *Contributions to a Pathography of the Musicians.* 1. Robert Schumann. *Conf. Psychiat.,* **2,** 65.

THE CREATIVE PERSONALITY*

Eliot Slater

The subject matter of my inquiry, is provided by a group of German musicians, some of them being among the greatest names the world has known. The questions which have been asked are about the relationship of personality to creative achievement. As I am a psychiatrist, the inquiry has been conducted along psychiatric lines. I am in all humility aware that the use of psychiatric weapons of research will not take us very far into the immense field that awaits investigation; but I believe that what the psychiatrist can contribute to the common pool of understanding is important and indeed essential. The title that I chose is intended to suggest that it is with the temperamental aspects of the creative worker that we shall be concerned tonight. The greatest and most central problems—What is the nature of artistic creation? What are the peculiar gifts of the genius in art?—these will have to be left almost untouched.

About twenty-five years ago, when I was working in a psychiatric research institute in Munich, I became acquainted with a Dr Adele Juda. She was working on the problem of the relationship of 'genius' to mental abnormality and mental illness. The term 'genius' is a useful one, but scientifically suspect. Juda, herself, did not make use of it. Instead, she defined the class of persons she wished to investigate, as all those people, speaking the German tongue, who had been in their own field the most gifted and creative of all born since the year 1650. She chose those whose mother-tongue was German, because she was going to be advised by German experts, and would not expect them to know the great men arising in other cultures as intimately as those arising in their own. She approached academic bodies, and men of known distinction in some specialist field, in order to get as authoritative a jury as possible. Each member of these juries was then asked to draw up a list of the

*From a lecture given at the University of Newcastle upon Tyne.

greatest men of the past, in their own line. Thus she had mathematicians to choose the great mathematicians for her, chemists to choose chemists, and musicologists to choose musical composers, etc. From the lists she obtained in each field, she could mark off the names which had been nominated unanimously, those who had been nominated only by a majority of assessors, and those who did not receive even a majority vote. These last were excluded, and were not further investigated. The assessors were asked to make their choice on a basis of achievement only, and to put out of their minds all extraneous considerations, such as whether the man could be called a genius.

This method of selection had the great advantage of containing no biases for which the investigator herself could be held responsible. It would be too much to say that it was altogether unbiased. As you will see, when I come to give you the names of the composers who were included in Juda's list, there are a few, such as Schoenberg, whose absence it is difficult to explain, except on the grounds that the assessors were unable to maintain a fully impartial judgement when faced with the more modern and revolutionary work. This, however, is beside the point insofar as the psychological make-up of the subjects of the investigation is concerned.

Juda accumulated a total of 294 persons, which she grouped into two main classes of 113 artists and 181 men of science. She investigated the personal histories of the subjects from the psychiatric point of view, and also their ancestry, their families and descendants. Her findings are, of course, statistical in nature. I shall not trouble you with more than two of them, which are of cardinal significance. She found that the incidence of psychosis, that is to say of the graver mental disorders, was only slightly greater than would have been expected from a sample of ordinary men; but that her subjects included a considerable number of abnormal personalities. Her technical term is 'psychopaths'; and by the criteria she used she could expect to find about 10 per cent of psychopaths in a random sample of the general population. Instead, she found among the artists 27 per cent, and among the scientists 19 per cent.

Now since ancient times, and especially since the time of Lombroso, it has been persistently maintained that the man of genius is mad or half-mad. This opinion is always supported by selected instances, that is, evidence of little weight; Juda's findings provide us at last with some reliable evidence, and its main weight is on the other side. We are shown that in a fair sample taken from the ranks of the most able and distinguished men the world has known, mental abnormality is indeed commoner than in the generality of mankind; but even then it remains true that the large majority of these great men are mentally normal, and suffer neither from mental illness nor abnormality of personality. This is not, at present, the fashionable view. Edmund Wilson, for instance, in his essay 'The wound and the bow', uses the legend of Philoctetes to state a case in an extreme form. Philoctetes was the one man who could avail to pull the bow and shoot the invincible arrow, and also the man who, because of a loathsome skin disease, was found intolerable by all the hosts of Greeks laying siege to Troy. The wound, says Wilson, is the price of the bow, the bow is the reward of the wound. Juda's work shows that this opinion is a superficial one; but her findings show a somewhat paradoxical state of affairs, which calls for further study.

Unfortunately Dr Juda died before she was able to see her book into print; and when it was eventually published, it was in an abbreviated form, without any case material. This seemed to me a scientific tragedy. I got in touch with the authorities in Munich, and by their great kindness was made a present of Juda's biographical material. It is hoped to analyse this material with a view to answering some important questions that Juda never touched on; and in view of their exceptional distinction, a beginning has been made with the German musicians. My colleague Alfred Meyer and I have worked together on this material, and have supplemented Juda's biographical information from English sources, trying to make it as complete as we easily can from the psychiatric point of view.

Juda had a total of 28 composers in her series, of which one has been omitted from our study as he is still alive. The names of the other 27 are: Handel, J. S. Bach, Friedemann Bach, Gluck, Stamitz, Haydn, Mozart, Beethoven, Weber, Marschner, Loewe, Schubert, Lortzing, Mendelssohn, Schumann, Liszt, Wagner, Franz, Bruckner, Cornelius, Johann Strauss the elder, Brahms, Hugo Wolf, Mahler, Richard Strauss, Pfitzner and Reger.

First just a few words about the incidence of mental disorders, that is the conditions which are sometimes called the insanities. Of these, Juda found only three. Gluck, after a healthy vigorous life, had a mental illness in old age which was caused by a succession of strokes. Hugo Wolf, and probably Schumann also, died of general paresis, that is a mental illness caused by syphilis. All these three, therefore, suffered from conditions which were essentially accidental in nature, and are in no way caused by any underlying instability of constitution. However, there are good grounds for thinking that, apart from his terminal illness, Schumann suffered from his youth on from recurrent depressive phases, of what the psychiatrist calls a manic-depressive type. One representative of illness of such a kind is not a heavy incidence, and I think we must pass these composers as, in this respect, a very healthy group.

The composers whom Juda regarded as psychopathic were Friedemann Bach, Bruckner, Gluck, Liszt, Mahler, Pfitzner,

Schubert, Johann Strauss, Wagner and Wolf. Dr Meyer and I have felt compelled to revise Juda's diagnoses, and would regard both Gluck and Schubert as normal, while including Beethoven among the abnormal. One might ask, how does the disagreement arise? One source is the appearance of fresh information. Surprising as it may seem, a good deal more has been learned on the factual side about Beethoven than was available to Juda. She did not have the advantage of reading the important work on Beethoven and his nephew by the Sterbas, which, with the aid of a great amount of documentary research, entirely disposes of the old idea that Beethoven's nephew was a young scoundrel who broke the heart of the grand old man. Instead, it seems clear that Karl Beethoven was quite an average young man, who led a fairly blameless life and stood by his uncle with remarkable love and loyalty; and that the accusations that Beethoven heaped upon his shoulders, including one that he was having incestuous relations with his aunt, arose from the suspicious temperament and jealous possessiveness of Beethoven himself.

The evidence for a rather extreme abnormality of personality in Beethoven is very full. For many years he lived in his own home in circumstances of unnecessary squalor. He continually changed his lodging, and never made a real home for himself. He quarrelled constantly with his servants, and thought that they all stole from him. He had a lifelong fear of poverty, and counted the halfpence in a penurious way.

He showed also a strong streak of sadism. Asked to play at a gathering, he said he would comply only if another well-known composer who was also present would crawl under the table on all fours—and the latter actually complied. Again, about a new servant he wrote 'if he is a little hump-backed, I shouldn't mind, because then one knows immediately what is his weak side to attack him on'. He pinched and even bit his aristocratic pupils, and wrenched the fingers of the Archduke Rudolf to pay him out for being kept waiting.

He was extremely suspicious all his life, and, for instance, in 1809 wrote that he was compelled to leave Vienna by intrigues and cabals and base actions of all kinds. He suspected his servants were secretly in the pay of his sister-in-law Johanna, the despised mother of the nephew he adored. In his last years he was having his wine and food tasted for him. At the dinner to celebrate the first performance of the IXth symphony, he accused his friends of falsifying the box office receipts and cheating him—so that they all got up and went out, and he was left to finish the banquet with Karl alone.

In addition he was totally self-centred, ruthless and inconsiderate, impulsive and lacking in self-control, a hypochondriac, a prude (the libretti of Mozart's operas were too lascivious for him), and shabby and at times unethical in his financial dealings.

If we adopt what I believe to be the best of all definitions of a psychopath, that is a man whose personality deviates far from the statistical norm, and in a way which causes either him or society to suffer, then Beethoven was certainly a psychopath. Whether his psychopathy was inborn, or whether it was rather a reaction to the tragedy of the deafness which came on him at the age of 28, is a question which need not here be discussed.

In the case of Schubert, the revision which we make in Juda's diagnosis is in the opposite direction, and again because of the availability of further evidence. Juda took the view, which was indeed the standard one at the turn of the century, that Schubert was an irresponsible bohemian, who composed, when he felt like it, by a turn of untaught genius, and for the rest spent his time in Viennese cafés overindulging in food and drink. He could not even apply himself to the earning of a regular income, and thought the state should pay him for doing his work of composition. This is the sort of personality which might go with the composition of such light-weight material as songs; and it seems that the popular idea of what Schubert's personality was like depended a good deal on his rating as an artist.

In a recent biography, Brown has pointed out the falsity of this view. With the modern estimation of his chamber music and symphonies, the magnitude of his work comes to be seen as of an entirely different order. Furthermore, there has been in recent years the discovery in the archives of unpublished manuscripts, of innumerable sketches and preliminary drafts of many of his more important works, showing that he did not dash them off, but put in a lot of plain hard work. Finally there came the collection and publication by Otto Deutsch of contemporary documents reflecting light on Schubert. From this it could be shown that Schubert was neither an alcoholic nor an irresponsible bohemian.

Reviewing the psychopathic personalities among the composers, we are left with the list: Friedemann Bach, Beethoven, Bruckner, Liszt, Mahler, Pfitzner, Johann Strauss, Wagner, Wolf. With nine representatives in a total of 27 composers, the list is undoubtedly a long one, and it is now incumbent on us to examine the question whether there is any causal relationship between abnormalities of personality and musical creativity. If we go to individual cases to see whether some particular character trait bears a relationship to working capacity, it is clear that we may find any one to three different connections. The individual may have been hampered by the character trait in question, but have succeeded in its despite; there may be no relationship between the trait and the working capacity; and finally the trait may have had some positive effect in furthering creative work. I think that the list of men at which we have arrived offers examples of all three states of affairs.

Wilhelm Friedemann Bach was regarded by his father, J. S. Bach, as the most talented of his sons and as gifted as himself. However, he did not have Johann Sebastian's solidity of character and was weak-willed and irresponsible. Most damaging of all, he was lazy, or at least lacking in energy and persistence. We call him a psychopath because in course of time he became unable to keep a salaried post, could not support his wife and children and, in effect, abandoned them, and ended his days in squalid circumstances. He failed also in standards of musical integrity, and on at least one occasion passed off work of his father as his own. Most biographers believe that he was alcoholic. On the creative side, he preferred to improvise; and the total amount of composed music he put to paper is relatively very small, though its quality and originality are recognized by musicologists. It seems quite likely that but for his defects of character, above all his incapacity for sustained work, he would have been a much greater figure than he actually is.

Another example is offered by Bruckner. Bruckner's psychopathic trait was obsessionality. He had a counting mania which came on him at times of fatigue or reduced physical health, and would stand counting the leaves of a tree or the windows in a town view. He had a preoccupation with death and corpses, and insisted on witnessing the exhumation of Beethoven's body. At the age of 42 he was off work for some months taking a cure for his nervous symptoms. But apart from this his whole life was passed in a search for security. He was always trying to pass examinations, and later in life to get himself a university degree. Redlich comments that his music is affected by his counting mania, showing itself in a partiality for stiff regularities of periodization, bringing him sometimes dangerously near to rhythmic monotony. To his obsessionality, also, one can refer his incapaity to satisfy himself with the completion of a work. In symphonic composition he could not content himself with the natural climax, but would have to go on to a second; and he would write and re-write successive versions of the same composition, without being able to let it go out of his hands. Here, too, we see a psychopathic character trait exercising, as far we can tell, a wholly one-sided and negative effect.

As an example of a neurotic symptom apparently having absolutely no bearing on creativity we may take the case of Johann Strauss. Strauss was troubled by numerous phobias. He had a fear of heights, and travelling through mountains would sit on the floor of the carriage, or draw the curtains so as not to see. When his house was on a hill, he had to be conducted up it; and he would drink champagne to fortify himself against the ordeal of crossing a viaduct in a train. He had a horror of death, would not have death spoken of in his presence. Trying for him as these symptoms no doubt were, it is not at all easy to see how they had any effect on his work. Incidentally, he is the only example in our group of a man troubled with anxiety symptoms; when one thinks how common the minor degrees of predisposition to anxiety are, this is a striking fact.

Conditions such as those mentioned, which have no positive effect on creativity, should be rarer in our group of composers than in the generality of mankind; and this seems to be actually the case with anxiety tendencies. If there are abnormalities of personality which further musical expression, then we should find them in relative abundance. There is a strong suggestion that this may be said of two such traits, the cyclothymic disposition and the hysterical disposition. Let us take the latter first: it is shown in some degree by three of our nine psychopathic composers, Liszt, Mahler and Wagner, but by the last of these to a superabundant degree.

Wagner fulfils our definition of a psychopath, since he was always in difficulty himself, for instance through his political activities and by his incorrigible habit of running into debt; and he caused difficulties to others by his ruthless exploitation of his friends. His hysterical disposition is shown in his extreme egocentricity, his tendency towards self-dramatization and his need to have a spotlight always playing on him. I take the liberty of quoting Ernest Newman:

> Publicity was as much a necessity to him as food and air. The most interesting person in the universe to him was always himself . . . [he had the need] of dominance for dominance's sake . . . Always there was the inability to conceive himself . . . except as the central sun of his universe . . . An actor he certainly is in many of his letters—an actor so consummate as to deceive not only his audience but himself . . . Wagner could never imagine any other motive for opposing him except (1) that the opponent was paid to do so or (2) that he was either a Jew or under the orders of Jews.

A characteristic episode in Wagner's life was the Wesendonck affair. At the time when he was engaged on *Tristan* the Wesendoncks invited Wagner and his first wife Minna to be their guests and live in a small house at the end of the garden of their more commodious mansion. It was not long before Wagner and Frau Wesendonck were engaged in a passionate love affair. Newman describes it in these terms.

> He is at work on *Tristan*. Frau Wesendonck is necessary to him if he is to maintain the artistic mood that the poem and the music require.

Everything and everybody must therefore give way to this great need. He is utterly and honestly unable to see the situation through either Otto's eyes or Minna's. The former he dramatizes also; of the grief the good man must have felt at seeing his wife's infatuation for a man who calmly took possession not only of the wife but of the whole household, he had plainly no conception. He allots Otto *his* part in the play: they are all playing parts, and the title of the tragicomedy is 'The Three Renunciators' . . . So colossal was Wagner's egoism that he could not realize the bare possibility of the affair taking on in other people's eyes any aspect but that it had for his own.

Wagner complained bitterly when his wife repeatedly took exception to the goings-on. Of an intrigue which involved secret letters and the giving of orders to servants to deceive their masters, Wagner could write: 'It would never be possible to make a nature like my wife's comprehend relations so lofty and unselfish as ours'.

It is understandable that the capacity for living oneself into a part, the personality trait that derives satisfaction from the exhibition of violent emotions, should show itself to advantage in the creation of productions for the stage, and to disadvantage in the management of day-to-day life. In one field, the artist has to be able to let himself go, whereas the greatest aid to successful citizenship is self-control. That trait of personality which lends a stagey quality to emotional expression in normal life may well be the same as one which brings a living quality into the stage scene. Emphasis of gesture and intonation, an application of greasepaint, look differently behind the footlights than in the light of day. In our group of composers, those whose creations for the stage achieve transcendance are Gluck, Handel, Mozart, Wagner and Weber, and of them three, Gluck, Wagner and Weber were gifted in this way. The parallelism between the manifestations of the personality in day-to-day life and in artistic creation in the case of Wagner can be brought out in two further quotations. Of the man his acquaintance Schure wrote:

> The frankness and extreme audacity with which he showed his nature, the qualities and defects of which were exhibited without concealment, acted on some people like a charm, while others were repelled by it. His gaiety flowed over in a joyous foam of facetious fancies and extravagant pleasantries; but the least contradiction provoked him to incredible anger. Then he would leap like a tiger, roar like a stag. He paced the room like a caged lion, his voice became hoarse and the words came out like screams . . . He seemed at these times like some elemental force unchained, like a volcano in eruption.

And of his music Newman writes:

Like Bach, Wagner could never conceive any emotion without intensifying it to the utmost. The barest hint of joy in one of Bach's texts will set him carolling like a lark; the barest hint of mortality will bedim his music with all the tears of all the universe for its dead. Wagner has the same insatiable hunger for expression. In *Tristan* in particular every emotion is developed to its furthest limit of poignancy. The passion of love became almost delirium; when Tristan, in the third act, sings of the thirst caused by his wound, our very mouths, our very bones, seem dried as if by some burning sirocco blowing from the desert; when the sick man praises Kurvenal for his devotion it is a cosmic paean to friendship that he sings.

Now the psychiatrist is inclined to see, in the transports of the hysteric, something not quite convincing, something that suggests insincerity. I think we may say that, in a work of art, any quality of the work which had this effect on the participator would be completely fatal to it. Wagner's music is, of course, not found to be universally faultless; but among the criticisms that have been made I have not yet seen any accusation of insincerity. If our interpretation of Wagner's psychopathic disposition as hysterical is correct, this is something of a paradox. Perhaps it may be explained.

The stagey and unconvincing quality of the emotional display of the hysteric in ordinary life is derived from the intuitive sense of the observer that to some degree there is more emotion shown than is actually felt, that the subject of observation is not involved in the totality of his personality but is himself observing, and controlling his own antics. From the accounts we have of Wagner's behaviour, such a thing as self-control was totally impossible to him. There was no part of him that was coolly observing and unconvinced. When he wrote of the unselfish and lofty nature of his relationship with Frau Wesendonck, beyond the comprehension of such lower creatures as his wife, that was something that he absolutely believed, without a particle of reservation. Lack of insight is taken to a level at which a new sincerity, that of the child or the animal, has successfully taken over.

We now have to turn to the second of the psychopathic traits which I believe is positively associated with creativity, the cyclothymic tendency. A few words of explanation of what is meant by this term are needed.

The majority of mankind are moderately equable in temperament, and their moods of joy or sadness, elation or depression, occur within a narrow span and are a natural consequence of the circumstances of the time. There are some, however, whose mood is constantly varying, and not from any external cause but from an internal biological rhythm for which a physical constitutional basis will almost certainly one day be found.

In the upswing there is abundant unflagging energy, spontaneous joy in life, swift flow of ideas, bodily well-being; in the downswing there is unhappiness, loss of power of enjoyment, loss of spontaneity, self-depreciation, slowing of thought and ideas, bodily malaise. Moods in either of these two directions may be of long or short duration, from hours to months or even years; and the individual so constituted may pass from one mood directly into another, or through an interregnum of normality, which may also be short or last for years. The highest peaks of this fluctuation may reach the height of mania, the lowest troughs the depth of melancholia. In the life history of any one man, most swings are of only moderate degree.

Now it is a well known fact that a high proportion of creative workers find that there are periods in life when they have more than usual productivity, others in which they are more or less sterile. The lay observer, and indeed the man himself, will be inclined to say that he was happy because he was working well, that he was unhappy because he could not work. This may sometimes by true, but sometimes it is quite certain that cause and effect should be placed the other way round.

A case in point is certainly that of Schumann. Throughout his life he had ups and downs of mood for which no external cause can be assigned, and he began to have them from about his twentieth year and went on up to the onset of his fatal illness. The upswings never reached any excessive height, but in his depressions he was low indeed. He was then troubled with a leaden melancholy, fears of illness or insanity, guilt and self-depreciation, and insomnia. During these phases he was totally incapable of creative work. Mostly they were of short duration; but during the year 1844, the year in which he had his thirty-fourth birthday, they lasted with short gaps for the whole of the year. Not a single opus number is allocated to that year.

An even more remarkable case is that of Hugo Wolf. The whole of his life consists in short bursts of almost phrenetic activity, separated by long periods of sterility. His phases of active creation lasted from two to six months, his phases of inactivity from two to thirty-six months. When he could not work he was miserable, when he could he was full of joy; but to my thinking the mood change is the primary one. Thus in depressed inactive phases he speaks of wishing for an early end, of wishing to hang himself on the nearest tree; the inhibition was such that he was not only unable to compose, he could not even write a letter; he covered himself with self-contempt and had a horror of his own past work. In such a mood he writes that he cannot conceive what harmony, what melody is, and that 'I begin to doubt whether the compositions bearing my name are really by me'. When the mood failed, the inertial momentum of working failed to carry him through; the completion of one *Liederbuch* was delayed for several years by a sudden failure of mood.

In an active phase, exactly the converse state held. His high spirits had a warm infectious quality, even though he might still be irritable or impatient. A friend wrote, 'who has not seen Hugo Wolf rejoice does not know what rejoicing is'. The ideas then poured in such richness that, as he himself notes, he had scarcely the time to note them down.

It is not surprising that Wolf has been repeatedly diagnosed as a cyclothymic, even as a manic-depressive. His case, however, is less clear than Schumann's, as his personality was as a whole a much more complex one.

Other representatives of the cyclothymic disposition in our group are Cornelius, Handel, Marschner, Reger, Schubert and Johann Strauss.

Of course both the cyclothymic and the other composers, who are not cyclothymic, are liable to moods of a normal kind; but it is probable that the melancholy which arises as a psychologically normal reaction does not have the inhibiting effect produced by the depression arising from a biological cause. Joy and sadness, and indeed the whole gamut of emotional colours, supply motivation and material for expression in musical creation. But the composers, such as Bach and Mozart, who are not troubled by primary mood swings, are able to maintain a steady output of work, without any prolonged period of sterility.

If we are to think of the cyclothymic disposition as being in some ways a useful trait to the creative artist, then this might be so for two reasons. Whereas the cyclothymic is rendered incapable of imaginative work in a well-marked depression, he has the compensation of finding such work exceptionally easy, of having his ideas flowing richly and abundantly, in the opposite phase. Furthermore, the cyclothymic man is generally an extravert, impressionable, with warm and strong emotions generally; and I think that everyone would agree that there is not such a thing as a major work of composition without a rich emotional content. A quality which distinguishes the composers as a whole from the generality of mankind is their capacity for strong and deep emotion; to use another Jungian classification of temperaments, they belong to the feeling rather than the thinking type.

One of the things that we noticed with the cyclothymic was that in his depressed phases vital energy was generally low; he was not only unable to compose, he might even be unable to write a letter. This energy is the life-blood of creation. The general model of development which the creative process follows starts with the nascent idea;

through a period of latency and incubation there is a gradual building up of tension, which breaks, with the onset of effective
expression, into a sustained flow of outpoured energy, in a high and
sweating excitement that goes on hour after hour. 'I work at a
thousand horse-power', said Wolf. For such a process to occur at
all, the personality must have a capacity for accumulating reserves.
Availability of resources of energy would seem to be a necessity for
work of any magnitude. It is, then, instructive to look at the
members of our group to see whether there is evidence to support
this view.

The composers can be divided into those who received
unanimous nomination by the assessors, and those who were
nominated only by a majority; we can for convenience take the latter
as having the lesser achievement. In the list of those unanimously
nominated we have: J. S. Bach, Beethoven, Brahms, Bruckner,
Gluck, Handel, Haydn, Mendelssohn, Mozart, Reger, Schubert,
Schumann, Wagner, Weber. In the second list, among less
distinguished names, we have Liszt, Mahler, Johann Strauss,
Richard Strauss and Hugo Wolf. If we look only at the mass of work
produced by the former, we find that it is much greater per man
than that produced by the latter. The difference is not only one of
quality, but also of gross quantity. This is not to deny that there is a
good deal of individual variation, but the class difference exists too.
As an example we may take the case of the two Bachs.

Johann Sebastian, the father, was creatively active throughout his
life. In addition he had onerous duties as teacher and choirmaster,
and he brought up a large family, himself doing a lot of the teaching
of his children, in Latin and general education as well as in music.
His son Friedemann, whose musical gifts his father thought equal
with his own, carried a much smaller burden of family
responsibility, but found even that too much. He could not be
bothered with the hard work of writing and scoring, and found even
routine musical duties a nuisance. Johann Sebastian was a broad-
shouldered powerfully built man, Friedemann was more slightly
built, with beardless face and large soft earnest eyes. If we rate the
composers by the amount of energy they displayed in general affairs,
then we find all the greatest names coming high up in the list.

Somewhat related to energy of personality, though essentially
distinct, is the quality of aggressiveness of combativeness. We find
this quality also well represented. J. S. Bach, Beethoven, Brahms,
Gluck, Handel, Mahler, Johann Strauss, Wagner and Wolf were all
extremely combative men; and their life stories contain dramatic
accounts of their struggles with administrative superiors, colleagues,
enemies and the world at large. However, there are as many lacking
this feature of personality; and, for example, such supremely

productive creators as Haydn and Mozart, though clearly well
endowed with energy, had no tendency to charge into battle against
the opposition.

Big men tend to be less energetic, and less combative, than men of
small stature. Unfortunately the necessary facts are not always
available; but I have been unable to learn of more than two
composers in our group who were of more than average height—
Gluck and Schumann. A few of the others are said to have been of
average height; but Brahms, Haydn, Liszt, Mahler, and
Mendelssohn were all less than average, Wagner was described as a
pocket edition of a man, and Mozart, Schubert and Hugo Wolf were
not more than one or two inches above five feet. These very small
men were also slenderly built, which was of no physical disadvantage to them—we know that a small and slender frame can be
compact of vigour. Most of the men of average height or more, were
in general strongly and solidly built. Schumann is the only one to
approach at all towards the loosely built, tall figure.

There is evidence to connect energy of personality with sexual
functions; and here we find to our surprise that quite a number of
the most dynamic and masculine of these men never developed any
permanent relationship with women. Beethoven, Brahms, Bruckner,
Handel, Schubert and Wolf never married. Schubert and Wolf
certainly had love affairs. Brahms is said to have amused himself
with chambermaids and women of easy virtue, and Handel to have
had affairs with his singers. Beethoven had an extraordinary attitude
towards women, varying ambivalently between the grossest
contempt and a sentimentalized reverence. One of the medical
theories of the cause of his deafness, and of the liver cirrhosis of
which he died, is that it was caused by syphilis. If that were true, it
would partially explain why, when he developed a tenderness for a
woman he could respect, his advances would at some point turn into
a hurried retreat. Of all the candidates for the garland of lifelong
chastity, Bruckner is the most promising. He was always fancying
himself in love and, indeed, trying to get married; but he was such
an awkward figure, and he managed his courtships so uncouthly,
that no woman would have him. However, Redlich in his biography
insists that normal physical relationships with women were not
unknown to him. On the physiologically deficient side, Haydn and
Reger made highly abnormal marriages, in which the sexual
element may have been weak or lacking. On the other hand there
are many who show evidence of more than average sexual vigour.
J. S. Bach married twice and had a very large number of children;
Loewe and Wagner were also married twice, Johann Strauss three
times, Marschner four times. Though Liszt never married, he had
two mistresses with each of whom he lived for many years, having

children by the first; and in addition he had innumerable love affairs of a transient kind. There is no doubt that three men, at least, were intensely susceptible to erotic emotion, Liszt, Johann Strauss and Wagner. How then are we to account for the celibacy of men of such dynamism as Handel, Beethoven and Brahms? This is not a matter on which biographers provide the medical psychologist with the physiological detail he would like to have; but it seems probable that their celibacy was not due to defective sexuality, but rather to a determination, conscious or unconscious, to maintain total personal independence.

We are now at last beginning to arrive at a kind of composite picture. The sketch is a very provisional one, and could do with a lot of filling in. In terms of temperament, these men depart from the average of mankind in having a greater capacity for feeling, for emotional reaction. Not only do they react to the environment in a more powerfully emotional way than most men, they also contain an excessive number of personalities of the cyclothymic kind, that is, subject to biological swings of mood. In addition, the personality is more than normally energetic, vigorous, even aggressive and combative. Despite their liability to a level of intensity of emotional reaction that the normal personality would be unable to tolerate, they are little liable to neurotic illness. I can find only four of them who ever sought medical treatment for their 'nerves': Bruckner took a three-months cure at a spa, for a depression, at the age of 43, Franz had a depressive reaction to going deaf, Liszt was off ill after an unhappy love affair at 16, and Loewe had spa treatment at 66.

By the term 'neurosis' or 'neurotic illness' the psychiatrist means a condition in which the sufferer complains of symptoms for which no physical basis can be found, and for which he comes to the doctor for help. This is, therefore, a state in which the personality admits at least a partial defeat. There may be physical symptoms, such as headache or dyspepsia, or nervous symptoms only—fatigue and weakness, worry and anxiety, obsessive compulsions or fears, depression, loss of memory or trances. It is incapacities of these kinds that we are liable to think of in connection with Edmund Wilson's wounded personality, which, he thinks, is the only one that can draw the bow. If we examine the abnormal personalities in our list, however, it is not this picture we see at all. With the exception of Friedemann Bach, none of these men were bleeding from an internal wound. They were not anaemic but full-blooded individuals.

Of the titanic energy of Wagner we have already heard; but we think also of Beethoven thrusting his way along a garden path through a crowd of courtiers, so that even the Emperor himself has to step out of the way, and murmur 'There have to be such people!'

We see Hugo Wolf, the almost unknown composer with all to lose, in his little column in the *Salonblatt* attacking Brahms, the then enthroned king of musical Vienna. The gentle Liszt did immeasurable things for the social standing of the executant artist, in fact creating such a position out of nothing, journeying up and down Europe in indefatigable tours. Though a snob, he did not hesitate to rebuke royalty itself when his playing was rudely disturbed by chatter, lifting his hands from the keys so that silence fell. When asked why he had stopped, he said with devastating politeness 'Music itself is silent when Ludwig speaks'. Mahler dominated his orchestra with an iron will that at last became intolerable to bear, though he raised the standard of performance to a point that Vienna had not known.

Such illustrations might be multiplied indefinitely. These men were not weaklings. Their abnormalities run rather to more positive, even if more objectionable faults of character—to arrogance, egoism, impatience, obstinacy, sensitivity and touchiness, irritable temper, ruthlessness and fanaticism.

How far are these grave faults accidental, one may ask, and how far germane? Certainly many of the greatest were free from them. But there is something in the life that must be led by the man with a gift to exploit that encourages the development of defensive attitudes which, out of their context, lead to difficulties. Such a man's first loyalty must be to the realization of his potentialities. Even such supreme egoists as Mahler and Wagner, who sacrificed the feelings of others to what looked like their private whims, again and again sacrificed their own interests, seen from the viewpoint of mere expediency, on the altar of what they took to be their destiny. With all his arrogance, the artist may still reserve for his own person a place of extreme humility. Of himself Hugo Wolf wrote: 'when the day comes that I can compose no longer, then no one should trouble himself about me any more; then they should throw me on the dung-heap; that for me is the end'.

WHAT HAPPENED AT ELSINORE
A DIVERSION

Eliot Slater

The following essay is offered as a tribute to all my friends who on other pages have brought their tributes to me. It is submitted to them in humility and gratitude, and with no ulterior wish than to entertain them. If in such a serious volume even such a frivolous piece as this must find its psychiatric justification, then let it point the moral of the inconclusiveness of all psychodynamic interpretation, however seemingly convincing.

Preliminary considerations

In recent years we have become confusedly aware that there is only a nebulous and shifting boundary between mythological and historical fact. We have had it explained to us that the founder of the Christian faith was a man only in the historico-mythological sense; mytho-historically, it was a sacred mushroom. Conversely, and to descend to a mundane level, it has been revealed that the picturesque personalities of Mr Sherlock Holmes and Dr Watson are more than merely fictional. Their life and times, under the intensive researches of Father Ronald Knox and his successors, have disclosed a core of hard facts that can be checked and counter-checked and inter-related down to the last detail. We must accept, without question, the mytho-historical reality of the ménage at 221b Baker Street. Visitors to London are regularly and very properly shown to the squares and streets frequented by Mr Pickwick and his circle. And who can seriously deny that life and reality belong to the personalities evoked for us by Marcel Proust in his researches into time past, rather than to their poor counterparts, whose pseudo-existence can still be traced in yellowing newspaper-files? In the year 1984, soon to be upon us, those of us who are then alive will be shown how historical reality is what you choose to make it. The past can indeed be abolished by deleting it from the records, and a new mytho-historical past can be written in.

Is this what Saxo Grammaticus did with his story of Amleth? It seems to me that he did, that he turned history into myth; and that if we want to reverse the process, and recover the mytho-historical reality, we must turn to the pages of Shakespeare. In the present context of Shakespearean research it would be absurd to suppose that Shakespeare was a mere man. He was, of course, not a man but a genius; which means that an immense range of learning was open to him without the need of education, and that he could command sources of factual knowledge by inspired divination. If we turn to Shakespeare, we can rely on him for the truth, the truth that is to say in an ideal sense, of everything he has reported. Let us for the moment abandon the trite and frustrating idea that in Shakespeare's *Hamlet* we are reading only the enactment of a play. Surely in our hearts we know that the castle and palace of Elsinore, whatever the Danes may say, was built on a lofty crag looking out over a grey and stormy sea; that in those chambers and antechambers, rooms and halls and corridors and narrow stairways, Hamlet and Gertrude, Claudius and Polonius, Ophelia and Laertes moved as creatures of flesh and blood, and through the tangle of plot and counterplot, treason and murder, poison and the sword, came to their tragic ends.

What is the truth that lies behind Shakespeare's complex narration, so inconveniently broken up into acts and scenes? Everything he tells us we must assume was true. Everything happened as he describes, but of course he describes not everything that happened. To fill these gaps we must use imagination and logic; and remember that, while Shakespeare always tells us the truth, the people he is telling us about, like all human beings, are often mistaken, and sometimes tell lies.

For example, Hamlet says things about Claudius which we cannot believe, things which clearly spring from his overmastering jealousy. Certainly, Claudius was no 'king of shreds and patches' (III.4). We know from the way in which he handles his court, how he deals with one emergency after another, how he copes with imminent danger of death at the hands of the insurgent Laertes, and how finally he does die, from all this we know that he was a man of resolution, endurance and fire. To captivate Gertrude we must think of him as a splendid figure of a man, regal in stature and bearing, handsome, courageous, passionate, for all his Borgia-like qualities. Hamlet's denigrations underline by their dramatic irony the calibre of his opponent.

Gertrude herself is such a woman as to inspire a passion that leads to adultery, fratricide and regicide. Hamlet tells us as much, *per contra*. 'At your age', he says to her, 'the hey-day in the blood is tame, it's humble, and waits upon the judgment' (III.4), which is what he wants to believe, and cannot; and with his help we see her, beautiful and sensual, with the eager blood pulsing in her arteries. She is a queen worthy of her king. In her reception of Rosencrantz and Guildenstern (II.2) her tart reminder to Polonius (II.2), and her sardonic comment on the Player-Queen, she shows herself capable of poker-faced mockery and an ironic wit.

How did King Hamlet die?

We come now to profounder questions, and the first is: did Claudius actually kill King Hamlet? Let us take the testimony of the Ghost (I.5). It was given out, it says, that 'sleeping in my orchard, A serpent stung me', but in fact:

> . . . sleeping within my orchard,
> My custom always of the afternoon,
> Upon my secure hour thy uncle stole
> With juice of cursed hebona in a vial,
> And in the porches of my ears did pour
> The leperous distilment, whose effect
> Holds such an enmity with blood of man,
> That swift as quicksilver it courses through
> The natural gates and alleys of the body,
> And with a sudden vigour it doth posset
> And curd, like eager droppings into milk,
> The thin and wholesome blood; so did it mine,
> And a most instant tetter barked about
> Most lazar-like with vile and loathsome crust
> All my smooth body . . .

The confession of Claudius (III.3) runs:

> O, my offence is rank, it smells to heaven,
> It hath the primal eldest curse upon't,
> A brother's murder!

Claudius certainly believed he had killed his brother; but the Ghost's story does not hold water. Hebona signifies henbane or hyoscyamus, of which the toxic principle is hyoscine. This is a sedative neurotropic drug, and is not a haemocoagulant, with effects such as those described in the Ghost's account of the symptoms. Moreover, it is an alkaloid, which can be assimilated into the body if swallowed, or injected, but cannot be absorbed through the skin, either of the external auditory meatus, or anywhere else. If Claudius actually killed King Hamlet, he must have used some other method. This does not seem likely. What seems more likely, in view of his reactions to the performance of The Mousetrap, is that Claudius attempted murder by the means described, and was a murderer in will and spirit; but that his murderous act was not the proximate cause of death. The symptoms described by the Ghost are in fact compatible with snakebite.

Whose ghost was it?
This brings us a stage further. Can anyone maintain that the Ghost is to be taken seriously? Does anyone believe that the ghosts of murdered kings, with their accoutrements of phantom armour, have ever been otherwise descried than by the strong eye of faith? Surely, in the events on the battlements, there is a suggestion of intervention by all-too-human agencies. This hypothesis explains many difficulties, including those that have been raised about Horatio. To quote Madariaga (1964, p 112):

> Many are the critics who have rightly observed that Horatio does not tally with himself. In some ways he is a stranger to the land, about which he asks obvious questions; in others, he seems to be one of the trusted courtiers of the King and Queen. He had come to the King's funeral, but does not meet Hamlet till two months later; he is a scholar who has just come from Wittenberg and yet he is the only Dane of the three on the stage who can explain the cause of Denmark's military preparations.

All this is readily explicable if we think of him as Hamlet's under-cover man, having, among his many tasks that of egging the people on in disaffection to Claudius and in their love for Hamlet. His cover personality is, indeed, that of the trusted courtier of the King and Queen; but he disappears for weeks together, not to Wittenberg but into the Danish underground. He does know everything that is going on; and he asks obvious questions to see just how much the others know. He was present at the King's funeral, but, of course, carefully kept away from Hamlet. When they meet, though no doubt they have been in contact, and have been hatching their plans, they pretend to have been long parted (I.2).

Let us try to reconstruct the sequence of events. With his hatred of his uncle, and his fury that the latter had 'popped in between th'election and my hopes' (V.2), Hamlet's suspicions that his father's death was other than accidental are quickly aroused. He draws Horatio to him in aid, and is soon thinking of using the highly troubled political and international situation to his advantage. So let his father's ghost walk the battlements, and start the rumours going! With his father's armour available to him, the masquerade comes easily to that freakish undergraduate mind. When in I.4 he is himself watching on the battlements with Horatio and Marcellus, and Horatio cries 'Look, my lord, it comes!', Hamlet takes his cue, and with a powerful address to the Ghost drives home the suggestion to the semi-hypnotized Marcellus. When his two companions try to restrain him, he runs—how bravely!—after the illusory ghost.

Then happens something curious and interesting, but also very natural. Endowed with his own share of superstition, he seems to hear the Ghost speak to him—and out come all the corrupting hates and fears and suspicions which he has been harbouring in his mind, some perhaps till now unconsciously. He is, momentarily but only momentarily, convinced of the veridical nature of the apparition.

He is recalled to his senses by hearing his followers calling for him. At once his spirits rise to a peak of delight in the prank he has played. He can hardly help himself from laughter. 'Hillo, ho, ho, boy! come, bird, come' he calls. 'It is an honest ghost', he tells them; and then there is a sudden change in his intentions. Instead of repeating the Ghost's accusations, as was probably part of the original plan, he swears his followers to silence.

What ensues is something that has never been adequately explained by the commentators. As he holds out his sword for them to swear on, the voice of the Ghost is heard from under, saying 'swear'. This is another piece of Hamlet's amateur theatricals, probably done impulsively, when it was not in the script at all. It is a neat act of ventriloquism. He is delighted with its success, and calls back to the 'Ghost'

Ha, Ha, boy! say'st thou so? Art thou there, truepenny?

and then to his followers:

Come on, you hear this fellow in the cellarage,
Consent to swear.

And so to an encore and a second encore of the same ventriloquial act, finally dismissing his supernatural stooge with

Well said, old mole! canst work i'th'earth so fast?
A worthy pioneer!

All this mummery leaves Hamlet in some real doubt whether by his own trickery he has not called up an actual spirit of the dead. He shows himself in two minds at later stages in the action; but in the closet scene, after the murder of Polonius, his unconscious breaks through again, and with hallucinatory vividness the dead father is seen and heard by him, but not, of course, by his mother.

The political crisis and the threat of war
We must now consider the political and international background at the time when Shakespeare's record opens. Marcellus (I.1) asks:

> Tell me who knows
> Why this same strict and most observant watch
> So nightly toils the subject of the land,
> And why such daily cast of brazen cannon
> And foreign mart for implements of war,
> Why such impress of shipwrights, whose sore task
> Does not divide the Sunday from the week,
> What might be toward that this sweaty haste
> Doth make the night joint labourer with the day . . .?

Horatio explains. A generation ago, at the time when Hamlet was born, Fortinbras of Norway had engaged in single combat with King Hamlet of Denmark, staking 'all those his lands/Which he stood seized of', 'Against the which a moiety competent/Was gaged by our king'. King Hamlet slew Fortinbras, and won his lands. It is not said so, but we must suppose that the land which Fortinbras lost was, not in the Norwegian but in the Danish peninsula, and that by the victory the territorial integrity of Denmark was established. Now, as the story opens, King Hamlet being dead, young Fortinbras, intent to avenge his father and recover the lost lands, has collected a volunteer army, and is threatening to invade Denmark. King Claudius himself confirms this (I.2), informing us also that Fortinbras has actually been making demands for the return of the lost lands.

Claudius writes to the King of Norway, who is old and bedridden and may not have appreciated what Fortinbras is purposing, to ask him to suppress his nephew's activities; and the Danish ambassadors depart charged with the delivery of this missive.

The diplomatic démarche succeeds in its aim. In II.2 the ambassadors return, and Valtemand reports. The King of Norway had understood that the levies raised by Fortinbras were to be directed against the Poles; but when he found that the campaign was to be against Claudius, he had Fortinbras brought summarily before him. Fortinbras is rebuked, and

> Makes vow before his uncle never more
> To give th'assay of arms against your majesty:
> Whereon old Norway, overcome with joy,
> Gives him threescore thousand crowns in annual fee,
> And his commission to employ those soldiers,
> So levied, as before, against the Polack,
> With an entreaty, herein further shown,
> That it might please you to give quiet pass
> Through your dominions for this enterprise,
> On such regards of safety and allowance As therein are set down.

Claudius replies 'It likes us well', and promises to think about it; permission *laisser passer* is accorded in due course.

So Fortinbras, in exchange for a paper promise (if indeed that was ever exacted) to proceed against Poland and not Claudius, receives his uncle's blessing, a plentiful exchequer, a royal commission, an official army—and safe-conduct into the heart of Denmark! It is an extraordinary affair. One feels inclined to suspect that the King of Norway, senile though he be, is not so witless as to perceive the chance of recovering, through the instrumentality of Fortinbras, lands that were previously Norway's. Is it possible that Fortinbras and his king have a secret understanding?

But the most amazing aspect of the affair is the infatuated behaviour of Claudius who, for no quid pro quo or other visible cause, allows the armed intrusion of a foreign power, an army under the command of a soldier who has proclaimed his hostility and his intention of wresting Danish lands into his own possession. Whatever his political abilities, Claudius is totally unfitted to be his country's commander-in-chief. He seems to have no idea of the most ordinary security provisions. Not only does Fortinbras with his army arrive at the end suddenly and unheralded at the Danish court, but even before that Laertes, at the head of a civilian rabble, has been able to overpower the palace guards, and take the king's person into his hands.

How was it that Claudius could agree to such a dangerous intrusion by Fortinbras? One suspects that he has been advised by his old counsellor and friend, Polonius, a statesman from whom one would expect a strategy of appeasement. But what of Hamlet? Has he any part in this? Claudius has the highest opinion of his abilities, as any thinking man would be bound to have, and calls him (I.2) 'Our chiefest courtier, cousin and our son', and wants, above all, to have him at his side. Is it possible that Hamlet has seconded Polonius in the policy of appeasement? And if so, what would his motive be? At this stage in the development of the situation at Elsinore he seems to have had no concrete plan in mind, but, rather, to be tortured by the need to formulate a plan.

Hamlet and Fortinbras

Hamlet's first preoccupation is to fathom the mind of the king, and to convince himself of his guilt. He does indeed succeed in this; but he is packed off to England before he can take any further open step. There now occurs one of those incidents which could be sheer accident, but which bear the strong appearance of the deliberate and resourceful use of a coincidence. As Hamlet traverses Denmark, under the guard of Rosencrantz and Guildenstern towards a suitable port, he crosses the path of Fortinbras and his army. Hamlet knows, of course, of Fortinbras, and of his projected route; he has his mind on a rendezvous. He meets the foreign army and from one of the captains of Fortinbras learns how flimsy is the pretext, the official pretext that is, for the campaign. Hamlet sees deeper. He dismisses the captain, and sends Rosencrantz and Guildenstern and his retinue on ahead. In the soliloquy that follows (IV.4) he reflects on the absurdity of a campaign involving the 'imminent death of twenty thousand men', and resolves:

> O, from this time forth
> My thoughts be bloody, or be nothing worth.

This is the last time he ruminates on his own vacillation. It is now, at last, that he begins to see his future clear ahead of him.

Hamlet sails for England, but encounters the pirates. In a letter, delivered to Horatio by sailors, Hamlet relates (IV.6):

> Ere we were two days old at sea, a pirate of very warlike appointment gave us chase. Finding ourselves too slow of sail, we put on a compelled valour, and in the grapple I boarded them. On the instant they got clear of our ship, so I alone became their prisoner. They have dealt with me like thieves of mercy, but they knew what they did. I am to do a good turn for them.

What, one wonders, did the pirates know? What was the bargain struck with them, and what good turn is Hamlet to do for them?

As many people have noticed, there is something very fishy about this story. Madariaga, who discusses it in detail, of course adopts the hypothesis which we have discarded, namely that we are concerned with a piece of fiction; but on that leaky bottom, he cannot make the story float. He writes (p 109):

> Events, as wild and unruly as a piratical attack is likely to occasion, are forced by the author to suit his plan so well that Hamlet and only Hamlet boarded the pirate ship and 'on the instant they got clear of our ship; so I alone became their prisoner.' As if this story was not tall enough the pirates turn out to be 'thieves of mercy', so that the plot could go on unmolested. All this is puerile and would not be tolerated in a modern author.

> But there is worse still. Hamlet says to Horatio that this sea fight took place the very morning after he had skilfully stolen the King's despatch from the baggage of Rosencrantz and Guildenstern and placed the changeling instead. It follows that Hamlet had acted thus in the expectation of arriving in England together with the two men he was sending 'to 't', since the pirates cannot have been so merciful as to have given him notice of their intentions. But what would have been the position then? The King of England would have received a 'command' from the King of Denmark to put to death two men in the suite of the Prince, heir of Denmark, who would do what?: profess to know nothing about it?—know all about it? The episode simply does not work; and everything in it goes to show that Shakespeare did not trouble to give any likelihood to that branch of possibility because

he—though not Hamlet—knew it would not 'happen', since he had in store a ship of pirates of mercy to bring Hamlet back. By way of consequence, the whole episode disintegrates.

Of course, once one recognizes that Shakespeare is telling us mytho-historical truth, Madariaga's argument breaks down. We can see why the pirates got away the instant Hamlet had boarded their ship, why they were thieves of mercy, why Hamlet knew he would never have to face the King of England with an unexplainable commission from his overlord of Denmark. We see how the plan was worked out.

After sending Rosencrantz and Guildenstern ahead, as related in IV.4, Hamlet hurries after Fortinbras, and, in secret conclave, comes to an agreement with him by which Fortinbras will recover the lost lands in exchange for help in deposing Claudius, bringing him to trial and execution, and setting Hamlet on the throne of Denmark. Rejoining Rosencrantz and Guildenstern and his retinue, Hamlet embarks. One of the ships of Fortinbras is detailed to follow Hamlet's, and when it is two days out to sea, to close with it, and rescue him. Hamlet is fully prepared for everything that follows, and for swift action in the emergency. He makes his dispositions for the welcome of his two attendants when they arrive in England; and is on the deck ready to leap abroad the pirate the instant the two ships close. After the rescue, when he is set again on Danish soil, he hurries to Elsinore, to meet an appointment with Fortinbras, and to prepare the final denouement. In the meantime Fortinbras, proceeding towards Poland, never actually leaves Denmark, but makes an abrupt turn, and by forced marches arrives suddenly and unannounced at Elsinore only a few hours after Hamlet.

No wonder that it is a wholly transformed Hamlet that we meet in Shakespeare's Act V, one who is now calmly confident of finishing his business with the King. Horatio reminds him.

> It must be shortly known to him from England What is the issue of the business there.

And Hamlet replies:

> It will be short, the interim is mine,
> And a man's life's no more than to say 'One' . . .

The tragedy of Ophelia

To come now to the key problem of the whole story—what is the matter with Hamlet?—we have first to ask, what is it ails Ophelia?

There are those who think of Ophelia as a maiden pure and undefiled; but Ophelia's chastity is one of the moot points of Shakespeare's narrative. In I.3 Laertes, her brother, warns her of the danger that she might allow herself to be seduced by Hamlet:

> Then weigh what loss your honour may sustain
> If with too credent ear you list his songs,
> Or lose your heart, or your chaste treasure open
> To his unmaster'd importunity.
> Fear it, Ophelia, fear it my dear sister,
> And keep you in the rear of your affection,
> Out of the shot and danger of desire.

Polonius, her father, loses no time in taking up the same issue:

> 'Tis told me he hath very oft of late
> Given private time to you, and you yourself
> Have of your audience been most free and bounteous
> If it be so—as so 'tis put on me,
> And that in way of caution—I must tell you,
> You do not understand yourself so clearly
> As it behoves my daughter and your honour.
> What is between you? give me up the truth.

The family are obviously alarmed by Ophelia's behaviour. Polonius goes on:

> Do you believe his tenders as you call them?
> . . . think yourself a baby
> That you have ta'en these tenders for true pay
> Which are not sterling. Tender yourself more dearly,
> Or (not to crack the wind of the poor phrase,
> Running it thus) you'll tender me a fool.

—That is, present me with a baby. He ends by saying:

> I would not in plain terms from this time forth
> Have you so slander any moment leisure
> As to give words or talk with the Lord Hamlet.
> Look to't I charge you, come your ways.

Ophelia says, compliantly 'I shall obey, my lord'. And the fact that she puts up no defence or objection suggests that she intends to 'go her ways', whatever the family says.

The next event is that Ophelia has a very frightening scene with Hamlet, and comes running to her father to tell him about it. We shall have to return to this later.

Then comes the 'nunnery' scene (III.1). After the most famous of all his soliloquies, Hamlet looks up to see Ophelia, and to say:

> Soft you now,
> The fair Ophelia—Nymph, in thy orisons
> Be all my sins remembered.

Is he not saying, almost in so many words, that his sins are her sins too? There follows a painful scene in which, from a very low and dejected state, Hamlet works himself up into an absolute rage. His sins, her sins, he cannot bear to think of them. Her beauty has betrayed him, 'for', he says, 'the power of beauty' (that's her) 'will sooner transform honesty from what it is to a bawd, than the force of honesty' (that's him) 'can translate beauty into his likeness'. 'Get thee to a nunnery' (that is, a brothel), he says, 'go, farewell . . . Or if thou wilt need marry, marry a fool, for wise men know well what monsters' (that is, men with horns, cuckolds) 'you make of them: to a nunnery, go, and quickly too, farewell'. He rushes out, but dashes back again, to sling more insults:

> I have heard of your paintings too, well enough. God hath given you one face and you make yourselves another, you jig, you amble, and you lisp, you nickname God's creatures, and make your wantonness your ignorance; go to, I'll no more on't, it hath made me mad.

He leaves, and Ophelia is left very cast down. She calls herself 'of ladies' (not 'of maidens', we notice) 'the most deject and wretched'. 'O, woe is me!' she says 'T'have seen what I have seen, see what I see'. The reversal of his passion from love to rage upsets her very much, but only for a short space, since it is but a little later that Hamlet is jesting with her in a very bawdy way at the play scene.

This passage is an important one, since it shows that she is so much in love as to be prepared to forgive him practically anything. The conversation is going on sotto voce, and Ophelia seems to find amusement in Hamlet's smutty remarks, 'That's a fair thought to lie between maids' legs', and the like. My own feeling, however, is that she is more delighted to be receiving notice again than tickled by the bawdry. However, there is no mistaking the mood of the following exchange:

> *Ophelia:* You are as good as a chorus, my lord.
>
> *Hamlet:* I could interpret between you and your love, if I could see the puppets dallying.
>
> *Ophelia:* You are keen, my lord, you are keen.
>
> *Hamlet:* It would cost you a groaning to take off mine edge.

This unabashed allusion to the act of love delights Ophelia: 'Still better—and worse', she says.

After the play scene occur the events which deprive Ophelia of everything that life held for her. Hamlet has killed her father; and he, her lover, her one hope of support, is exiled to England. Her brother is in Paris; and she is left utterly alone. Some think that she is aware that she is pregnant; but even if she is spared this, her life is in ruins. Ophelia's so-called madness is keenly observed and described by Shakespeare. It is what one would call a catastrophic depressive reaction, which becomes increasingly coloured by hysterical confusional and dissociative symptoms. Guilt lies heavily upon her soul—guilt, we may note parenthetically, lies heavily on the souls of all the major characters with the exception of Polonius. Somehow she must confess. Here we see the irony of events, for it is her occulted guilt which is unkennelled in one speech, and not that of Claudius. She enters the queen's apartments, carrying a lute, to which she sings (IV.5):

Tomorrow is Saint Valentine's day,
   All in the morning betime,
And I a maid at your window
   To be your Valentine.
Then up he rose, and donned his clo'es,
   And dupped the chamber door,
Let in the maid, that out a maid
   Never departed more.

She takes a breath, summons up her resolution, and says 'I'll make an end on't':

By Gis and by Saint Charity,
   Alack and fie for shame!
Young men will do't, if they come to't,
   By Cock they are to blame.
Quoth she, Before you tumbled me,
   You promised me to wed.
He answers:
So would I ha' done, by yonder sun,
   An thou hadst not come to my bed.

Now it is all out. 'I hope all will be well', she says and, in a moment or two, takes her leave: 'Good night, ladies, good night, sweet ladies, good night, good night' on her way to the night that has no ending.

What were the causes of Ophelia's ruin? What kind of childhood can she have had, what adolescence? She has lost her mother, about whose character we can only learn by implication, and, perhaps, lost her at an early age. What sort of a family was it, in which she grew up? Her brother, the noble Laertes, combines a quite remarkable number of detestable characteristics: he is a villain, a fool, a braggart, a libertine and a prig. In I.3 he takes it upon himself to preach a sermon to his sister, on the theme of 'ware Hamlet, and more generally,

The chariest maid is prodigal enough
If she unmask her beauty to the moon.

Ophelia knows just how much this is worth, and tells him:

But good my brother
Do not, as some ungracious pastors do,
Show me the steep and thorny way to heaven,

Whiles like a puffed and reckless libertine
Himself the primrose path of dalliance treads,
And recks not his own rede.

After that he is off to Paris; and his father knows what kind of life he can be expected to live there, namely gaming, drinking, fencing, swearing, drabbing and the frequentation of brothels.

We next meet him breaking in on King Claudius at the head of a rabble. He has the king in his power, and needs only the will and the hardihood to depose Claudius and ascend the throne. Instead of that he is promptly disarmed and set at naught; his furious enquiries are deflected by sophistries; in the space of a few minutes Claudius has converted him into his tool. The grave scene, which follows, is an abomination, with Hamlet behaving no better than Laertes; both of them have a fit of hysterics. In the last scene of all, of course, Laertes unmasks himself as a cold-blooded murderer.

Such was Ophelia's brother. And what of her father? In I.3 he discharges a load of wise saws on his departing son, lectures Ophelia on her chastity, and forbids her to see Hamlet again in private. In II.1 he is sending his agent Reynaldo to Paris to spy upon his son; it seems he has no strong objection to dissolute ways, but will want to know all about them. Later we see him pompous, garrulous and verging on senility, servilely swallowing every kind of insult Hamlet chooses to confer on him, but full of cunning, suggesting sly plans, hiding behind the arras to spy. No pedantry is too threadbare for him, no servility too slimy, no chicanery too pettifogging.

Hamlet, of course, loathes him and abuses him unmercifully. Moreover he makes a specific accusation. In II.2 Polonius unfolds to the king and queen his little ruse to trap Hamlet:

Polonius: You know sometimes he walks four hours together here in the lobby.

Queen: So he does indeed.

Polonius: At such a time I'll loose my daughter to him.
Be you and I behind an arras then . . .

What kind of a father is it, who 'looses' his daughter to the suspect? Hamlet comes in soon after, and very likely has overheard Polonius's little plan. The following conversation takes place:

Polonius: How does my good Lord Hamlet?
Hamlet: Well, God-a-mercy.
Polonius: Do you know me, my lord?
Hamlet: Excellent well, you are a fishmonger.
Polonius: Not I, my lord.
Hamlet: Then I would you were so honest a man.

Polonius: Honest my lord?
Hamlet: Ay, sir, to be honest as this world goes, is to be one man picked out of ten thousand.
Polonius: That's very true, my lord.
Hamlet: For if the sun breed maggots in a dead dog, being a good kissing carrion . . . have you a daughter?
Polonius: I have, my lord.
Hamlet: Let her not walk i'th'sun. Conception is a blessing, but as your daughter may conceive, friend look to't.

Fishmonger signifies bawd, and fishmonger's daughter means prostitute. Although Polonius is too thick to catch his drift, Hamlet is telling him that he, Hamlet, is aware of his game, aware that he is a proposing to use his daughter as a decoy and a catspaw. More, he is telling him that his daughter is a loose woman, a trollop, who may be pregnant in no time at all. Still more, he seems to be accusing Polonius of being a pander who has prostituted his daughter.

Has he? It is not unthinkable that this greasy old man, for the hope of advantage, could have done no less; such practices were a commonplace in the courts of Europe of the time. However, there are reasons for thinking that this is not what is in Hamlet's mind; this is not the low and vulgar intrigue that actually occurred.

In her confession, Ophelia makes it quite clear that it was she who, out of her lovesickness, and knowing no better, went to Hamlet's room, and that there she lost her virginity under promise of marriage. Now both her father and her brother thought that a marriage to Hamlet was out of the question. Both of them show themselves anxious about her relations with Hamlet, both of them suspect her of entering on a liaison, and for both the prospect is a cause of great apprehension. So it wasn't Ophelia Hamlet had in mind.

Why then should he call Polonius a fishmonger? If we consider the character of Polonius, particularly in the context of a small European court, we see that this pretentious wiseacre, this cunning fool, bears every mark of the cuckold. He was indeed born to wear the horns. Surely no woman could live with him, especially in such a court, without feeling compelled to make a fool of him. One conjectures that there have been stories circulating round the court for years. Hamlet has them in mind, and, making a glancing allusion to the misuse of his daughter, is reminding Polonius of having been a salesman of the favours of women professionally, as a part of his calling, having, in his time, bartered his own wife for advantage.

This surely is known to Laertes. In IV.5 he is making a great scene, but from beneath the braggadocio come up the thoughts festering in his mind to inflame to protest and denial. He shouts:

That drop of blood that's calm proclaims me bastard,
Cries cuckold to my father, brands the harlot,
Even here, between the chaste unsmirched brows
Of my true mother.

He too, like Ophelia, has a family skeleton to reveal, a confession to make, in his own way.

Ophelia's family, then, was not one to inspire in her any respect. She was, no doubt, drilled in etiquette and courtly observances; but from that family she could not have gained any lofty standards of behaviour, nor that self-respect and certainty of her own worth which gives the spirit fortitude when great troubles come. She falls for Hamlet hook, line and sinker; knows no better than to offer herself to him; and then finds herself first betrayed, then bereaved, and finally abandoned. Ophelia's tragedy is that of the innocent but unguarded soul in a decadent and corrupt court. At the very beginning of Shakespeare's narrative we are told there is something rotten in the state of Denmark; and we can be sure that it has been rotten, not for a month or two but for many years, to reach the depths at which the queen herself enters into an adulterous affair with her brother-in-law.

The tragedy of Hamlet

If we accept this solution of the problem posed by Ophelia, we come better armed to elucidate the more fundamental problems which confront us in Hamlet himself. In all the earlier stages of the action we find him melancholic, cynical, full of distrust and contempt for all his fellow creatures. More than all that, he is obsessed by a sense of personal worthlessness, personal and, specifically, sexual sin:

O, that this too sullied flesh would melt,
Thaw and resolve itself into a dew . . .   I.2

O, what a rogue and peasant slave am I!   II.2

A stallion! fie upon't! foh!   II.2

I could accuse me of such things, that it were better my mother had
not borne me: III.1

What should such fellows as I do crawling between earth and
heaven?   III.1

There is, indeed, something lying heavily on his conscience. Now, with regard to most of the seven deadly sins, his conscience is iron-clad. 'I am very proud, revengeful, ambitious' (III.1), he says, and clearly rather glories in these faults. He is apt for intrigue, ruthless and merciless. After the casual killing of Polonius, the father of the girl who loves him, he expresses no pang of regret. Dragging back the arras, he addresses the still twitching corpse (III.4):

> Thou wretched, rash, intruding fool, farewell!
> I took thee for thy better, take thy fortune,
> Thou find'st to be too busy is some danger.

And later, he says, as if the dead man were so much carrion:

> I'll lug the guts into the neighbour room.

Similarly (V.2) he confesses, without compunction, to having sent Rosencrantz and Guildenstern to their deaths, apparently for a mere whim, since no serious purpose can be divined. 'Not shriving time allowed', he adds; that is, if he is not an atheist, as he well may be, condemning them, one time his intimate friends, court parasites, if you like, but ones who have never done him any harm—condemning them to eternal fires. 'Why, man,' he says to Horatio (V.2):

> they did make love to this employment,
> They are not near my conscience.

Baldly stated, Hamlet is a triple murderer, in the end a five-fold killer. As far as action goes, he out-slays both Claudius and Laertes, and all without a qualm.

But there are things that make his skin crawl, and these are all the human functions comprised under the general category of sex. Obscenities are constantly in his mouth. For Hamlet's puritanical soul, sex is filthy, degrading, sub-human. But, being a man, he knows, all-too-personally, the prickings of the flesh.

Madariaga has justly commented that we cannot understand the action of Shakespeare's narrative without finding a key element in Hamlet's egocentricity (p 105): 'Hence his soliloquies. For, in fact, Hamlet soliloquises throughout the whole play. Whomsover he seems to be talking to, Hamlet only speaks to Hamlet'. This is very much the case when he is talking to his mother. When he is lashing at her, he is lashing himself. It is from the depths of his own carnal imaginations, his own carnal experiences, that he comes up with the obscenities with which to belabour her:

> Nay, but to live
> In the rank sweat of an enseamed bed
> Stewed in corruption, honeying, and making love
> Over the nasty sty—   III.4

His mother begs him to stop, but back he comes:

> Let the bloat king tempt you again to bed,
> Pinch wanton on your cheek, call you his mouse,
> And let him for a pair of reechy kisses,
> Or paddling in your neck with his damned fingers . . .   III.4

Hamlet's obsession with his mother's sex life is an overflow from his obsession with his own. It is his own honeying and making love, his own paddlings and reechy kisses which make his stomach heave. We can see now what a terrible wound it was that Ophelia dealt his self-pride when she insinuated herself into his bed. Maybe that early morning it was not only she who lost her virginity, but he also.

But this was a wrong that, one would suppose, could have been put right. Hamlet, the heir presumptive to the crown, could not have expected to pass his life in celibacy. Marriage would be an obligation, and he could have regularized his liaison with Ophelia, one would have imagined, with universal approval. To be sure she was not of royal rank; but she belonged to the nobility, and it would not have been an impossible misalliance. This was indeed the marriage which was hoped for by the queen his mother. At Ophelia's interment she says, scattering flowers:

> Sweets to the sweet. Farewell!
> I hoped thou shouldst have been my Hamlet's wife:
> I thought thy bride-bed to have decked, sweet maid,
> And not have strewed thy grave.

But there was a bar to the marriage, a secret bar, known, it seems, only to Ophelia's intimate family, though not to her herself. It was this that lay heavy on the minds of her father and her brother, and this it was that set Hamlet out of her star.

Now I must take you back to the very strange scene, which is the only evidence the commentators can claim that Hamlet was ever mad. We all accept, now, that Hamlet was mad in craft only, except for that one direction, north-north-west. This scene tells us what direction that was, how the compass points. Ophelia enters to Polonius (II.1):

> *Ophelia:*   O my lord, my lord I have been so affrighted!
> *Polonius:* With what, i'th'name of God?
> *Ophelia:*   My lord, as I was sewing in my closet,
> Lord Hamlet with his doublet all unbraced,
> No hat upon his head, his stockings fouled,
> Ungart'red, and down gyved to his ankle,
> Pale as his shirt, his knees knocking each other,
> And with a look so piteous in purport
> As if he had been loosed out of hell
> To speak of horrors—he comes before me . . .
>
> He took me by the wrist, and held me hard,
> Then goes he to the length of all his arm,
> And with his other hand thus o'er his brow,
> He falls to such perusal of my face
> As a' would draw it. Long stayed he so,
> At last, a little shaking of mine arm,
> And thrice his head thus waving up and down,
> He raised a sigh so piteous and profound

As it did seem to shatter all his bulk,
And end his being; that done, he lets me go,
And with his head over his shoulder turned
He seemed to find his way without his eyes,
For out adoors he went without their helps,
And to the last bended their light on me.

With all his disgust of sex, it is the thought of incest that, of all sins, most terrifies Hamlet. He cannot leave his mother's fault alone. Incest he calls it, again and again and again. But, observe he is the only one at court to miscall his mother's second marriage. The marriage of Claudius and Gertrude was officially solemnized by rites of Holy Church; and the state ceremony, which helped Claudius to the throne, was attended by the entire court. If, theologically, the union was incestuous, then there must have been ecclesiastical dispensation for it. Incest it was for Hamlet, for Hamlet only, and for his alter ego, the Ghost.

Now you have the answer to Hamlet's appalling sense of guilt. Now we know what were the 'foul crimes'—sexual misdemeanours, of course—that condemned the Ghost to walk the night. We know who the royal libertine was to whom Polonius prostituted his wife, and who it was that branded the mother of Laertes a harlot; what the secret was that, rankling in the breasts of her father and brother, all unknown to her, poor girl, set Hamlet out of Ophelia's star; whence sprang the thousand demons that clamoured 'Incest! incest! incest!' in Hamlet's tortured soul ever since, on a sudden discovery, rummaging in his father's private papers perhaps, the dreadful suspicion rushed in on him; and he burst into Ophelia's presence, the presence of the girl who had so innocently seduced him, to search her face for lineaments of resemblance, and to see there, alas, alas, his father's daughter, and his own blood-sister.

References

Madariaga, Salvador de (1964) *On Hamlet,* 2nd edn. London: Frank Cass.
Shakespeare, William (1968) *The Tragedy of Hamlet, Prince of Denmark* (Ed. John Dover Wilson) Cambridge University Press.

SOCIAL PSYCHIATRY

SOCIAL ANXIETY AND THE ROLE OF MEDICINE

E. H. Hare

Because of the success of the scientific method, the prestige of religion and magic has declined in industrial societies during the past three centuries. Many of the anxiety-relieving functions of religion and magic have been taken over by medicine. This is particularly apparent in the recent development of psychiatry which has assumed responsibility for the management of many conditions where distress arises much more from social than from physiological causes. It is argued here that medicine is in danger of becoming over-loaded by this new role. The development of non-medical modes of relieving social distress, as envisaged in proposals for a profession of psychotherapy, is likely to be the way in which the balance is redressed.

Individual and Social Anxiety
Anxiety is the instinctive response to an awareness that the future is uncertain and may be dangerous. In this broad sense, anxiety is natural to all animals and at its most basic level appears as a concern for where the next meal is coming from. With greater powers of foresight than other animals, man's concern for the future has extended to anxiety about ill health, pain and death. In addition, man as a social animal has another source of anxiety. He cannot exist—certainly cannot exist comfortably—except as a member of a social group and so he is exposed to anxieties about his membership of the group or of his status within the group. I suggest it is useful to think of everyone as exposed to two types of anxiety: *individual* anxiety, which concerns his bodily health and wellbeing; and *social* anxiety, which concerns his relations with his fellow men.

Up to a certain level, anxiety acts as a spur to effort but beyond that level it becomes increasingly unpleasant for the individual and, if severe enough, impairs his efficiency as a member of the group. We may presume that this is why every society has established systems for the relief of anxiety. My purpose in the present paper is to recall the ways in which anxiety-relieving systems have been organized and to discuss the part which the medical profession plays and ought to play in these procedures. From the priest *cum* medicine-man *cum* sorcerer of the primitive tribe, the three formal anxiety-relieving systems of civilized societies may be traced. These are religion, medicine and magic. Consider the state of these systems in Britain during the early part of the seventeenth century, a state which has been learnedly and delightfully described by Keith Thomas (1971) in his book *Religion and the Decline of Magic*.

Religion, medicine and magic

Religion was an institution primarily concerned with the cohesion of society. One of its functions was to reassure the general mass of people that those who seemed likely to rock the social boat by uncustomary behaviour would be the subject of its official disapproval. For those erring sheep who, consciously or unconsciously, strayed from the path of rectitude, religion provided the means of relieving their anxiety by welcoming them back into the fold on condition they repented their sin. Thus the anxiety-relieving procedures of religion were concerned with general anxieties about the stability of the group and with personal anxieties about membership.

Medicine was—and always has been—primarily concerned with the prevention and cure of bodily ill-health and with the relief of the pain and disability that may go with it. But as a sick person is very generally anxious for his life and wellbeing, medicine has also concerned itself with the relief of this natural anxiety, even when this arose not from any actual illness but from a fear of illness or from wrong ideas about the consequences of an illness.

Magic differed from religion and medicine in two ways. Magic worked by *spells* and a spell is a procedure designed to coerce the forces of the universe to produce the kind of future you want; whereas religion worked by prayer and sacrifice, procedures designed to persuade and entreat whatever gods there be. The second difference was that religion, and medicine too, were part of the Establishment and both had the very general approval of the most powerful members of society, whereas magic was officially considered disreputable and much of its practice was illegal. To intelligent people who become rather bored with the conventions of society, there is something very tempting in dabbling with matters on the fringes of good taste and the law. One of the great attractions of magic as an anxiety-relieving procedure was that its exponents were lone practitioners and, unlike the practitioners of medicine and religion, were not open to the suspicion that their practice was influenced by a corporate wish to maintain professional standards and income, or by an awareness that these depended upon a privileged position in the Establishment. You could consult a magician without fear that he would disapprove of you on legal or moral grounds or that his case records would be subpoenaed by a court of law.

The cure of souls and the cure of bodies

Each of the three great anxiety-relieving systems of society may be thought of as concerned with a particular type of anxiety: religion with anxiety about membership of the social group, medicine with anxiety about illness and death, magic with anxiety about social status and the achievement of ambition. In practice of course there was—and no doubt always has been—a good deal of overlap. One indicator of the overlap between religion and medicine is the different meanings given to the word 'health'. Etymologically, the word comes from the root meaning to make whole and is cognate with the word holy—holiness being a state of religious health. In the General Confession of the Prayer Book, we say that we have done that which we ought not to have done and there is no health in us; in modern times, on the other hand, medical authorities have argued that health has no social component (Lewis, 1953). The same division of meaning occurs in the word 'cure': the cure of souls is the business of a curate; the cure of bodies, of a physician. Such double usage lies in the fact that the distinction between religious (or social) health on the one hand and medical (or individual) health on the other is often a matter of opinion and dependent on the current fashion and state of knowledge. This is reflected in the history of witchcraft which was considered by most people in the seventeenth century to be a moral disorder—in other words, a state of wickedness or sinfulness. During the next three centuries, medical knowledge increased and opinion has veered to the opposite—and perhaps equally one-sided view—that those persons who had been called witches were really suffering from depressive illness or paranoia. Again, on the religious view, 'possession' was a state in which the devil entered into a person and took over his will, while 'obsession' was the state in which the devil sat down beside a person tempting him; and in each case, the person's soul might be cured by religious rites such as exorcism. Now, of course, we think of delusions and compulsions as medical matters, and though the evidence for their being due to derangements of bodily function is not really all that strong, most doctors believe that they can be, or will be (given time and research), curable by medicines.

Medicines and magic have always had a great deal in common. This is partly because both have their origins in what common folk called 'learning'. Doctors of all sorts were by definition learned, for only a learned person can teach; while to an Elizabethan—we have it on the authority of John Aubrey—the terms astrologer, conjurer and mathematician all meant the same thing. It is of course from this learned aspect of magic and medicine that what we now call science has developed. Yet until quite recently, the word science simply meant a formal body of knowledge; and a university distinction was made between the *natural* sciences (e.g. physics, chemistry, physiology) and the *moral* sciences (psychology, philosophy, theology). It is only recently that the term *science* has come to imply knowledge based on experimentally refutable hypotheses. In this restricted sense, only a small part of medical knowledge is scientific; and much of what is still called 'medical science' is science only in the sense of being part of a corpus of learning and belongs properly to the old moral sciences.

Apart from their common basis in learning, medicine and magic overlapped in their concern for many causes of human distress— impotence and infertility are among the most obvious—which are not moral in nature and which are not obviously due to ill-health. These were conditions for which medicine knew neither cause nor cure, and whenever this was so then medicine and magic were in competition to provide comfort and relief from anxiety.

Even today, medicine still hardly knows a cure for impotence or infertility, and it is a matter of common observation that these conditions will lead even the most educated persons to resort to charms and magic.

The declining prestige of religion and magic

Thus in one guise or another, the anxiety-relieving systems of religion, medicine and magic are always present but their circles of action overlap. The point I want to make now is that the nature and extent of the overlap is changing all the time. Such changes have been particularly marked in western civilization during the past three centuries and the main reason for this probably lies in the decline of religion and magic—or rather in the decline of the prestige they had in their seventeenth century form. Their decline is primarily attributable to the rise of science which destroyed the world-pictures of religion as represented by the biblical story of creation, and of magic as represented by the Ptolemaic universe. The astronomy of Copernicus and Newton and the biology of Mendel and Darwin were probably less satisfying emotionally than the old beliefs which, like psychoanalysis today, were self-confirming systems; but the new systems had the ineluctable advantage of a practical pay-off. A romantic might still regret this change: for, as J. B. S. Haldane observed, the cautious statement, 'my find ings are not inconsistent with the hypothesis that . . .' sounds feeble compared with 'Thus saith the Lord'. But such cautious statements reflect an important aspect of the rise of science: a recognition that the future cannot be predicted with certainty but must be assessed in terms of probability. In 1660, the young Dr Thomas Wharton (of Wharton's duct) enquired of the Oxford astrologer Ashmole whether he would ever be elected a Fellow of the Royal College of Physicians. The aspiring physician of today would still like to know his chances but he would hardly expect anyone to give a definite yes-or-no answer to an eventuality of that kind.

The rise of science was only partly due to the deliberate investiga-tions of pure-spirited alchemists and natural astrologers. It depended as much on the general increase in prosperity which began in the seventeenth century and has continued ever since. By reducing people's general anxiety about their immediate future, prosperity enables them to tolerate uncertainty better. Instead of needing to rush to the comfort of some immediate explanation, however inadequate, for a bad harvest or an epidemic disease, they have the leisure and the calmness of mind to make a considered study. Necessity, as A. N. Whitehead said, is the mother of futile dodges; it is leisure which is the mother of invention.

Thus the prestige of religion and magic declined, and their importance as systems for the relief of anxiety declined too. We must now consider what happened to the anxiety-relieving functions of medicine.

The rising prestige of medicine

It can hardly be doubted that the prestige of medicine has been increasing steadily since the time of William Harvey. Part of this increase must be attributed to the increasing role of science (in its modern sense) which, through the development of physiology and pathology, has lent its prestige to medicine as a whole. In addition, and whether due to scientific method or not, medicine had a series of spectacular achievements during the late eighteenth and the nine-teenth centuries—vaccination for smallpox, sanitation to prevent cholera and typhoid, anaesthetics, and the bacterial cause of many common diseases. Yet, except perhaps for vaccination and anaesthetics, the direct impact of these on the actual practice of medicine was probably slight. Even as recently as 1940, when I was a medical student, Sir Thomas Lewis could tell us that there were only four drugs of any real value in medicine—morphia, aspirin, digitalis and insulin. The prestige of medicine really increased, I suggest, for other, less obvious reasons.

During the whole of the nineteenth century there was a steady betterment in the general health of the population of Britain. One index of this was the continued fall in mortality rate from tuberculosis—a fall which is apparent from the time records began in 1840 and which has continued to the present day. There were minor reversals during the two world wars but the downward slope of the line was not noticeably influenced by the introduction of the anti-tuberculous drugs in the late 1940s. Cheaper and more plentiful food, cheaper and better clothing, warmer homes, smaller families (reflecting the introduction of contraception)—these no doubt were the major factors in the improvement in health. Medical knowledge, as expressed in sanitation, better understanding of the principles of nutrition, and wider provision of antenatal and obstetric care, no doubt played a part but probably only a minor part (McKeown, 1971). It is worth noting that an improvement in the general health of children means, when those children grow up, improved maternal health and so a further improvement for that reason in the health of the next generation of children; there is thus a virtuous spiral of healthiness. Now it is perfectly clear to a historian that the prestige of medicine can never have lain in its ability to cure disease. We have only to look at the old pharmacopoeias with their bezoar stones and crushed millipedes to appreciate this (millipedes were not deleted from the Edinburgh pharmacopoeia until 1803). The prestige of medicine has depended on its anxiety-relieving functions. Of course, patients are always ready to attribute their natural recovery to their doctors' efforts but that is understandable in terms of a wish to believe that someone knows the answer. In a period when general health is improving, and the *vis medicatrix naturae* is therefore stronger, more people will increasingly recover from illnesses and this circumstance will redound to the credit of the medical profession. I think this is probably the largest single reason for the increased prestige of medicine during the last 150 years. The process may still be continuing. Thus the prognosis of the functional psychoses has considerably improved during their last 40 years, and although this is generally attributed to advances in psychiatric treatment and therefore has added prestige to psychiatry, it seems just as likely to be due to a general improvement in constitutional health and a consequent greater resistance to disease processes of all kinds.

Scientific and non-scientific medicine
During the past three centuries then, the anxiety-relieving functions of religion and magic have suffered a decline, and those of medicine have increased. What are the consequences for medicine today? We might surmise that medicine will have taken over some of the

anxiety-relieving functions traditionally exercised by religion and magic; and it is this surmise which I now want to examine.

Present day medicine—in which I include psychiatry—is a mixture of the scientific and the non-scientific. Scientific medicine, in the strict sense, is based on refutable hypotheses and on objectively verifiable evidence: therapeutic efficacy must be examined by the method of controlled trial, and subjective evidence or impression, however authoritative, has little place. Non-scientific medicine is primarily concerned with the relief of the anxieties that may be associated with ill-health or the fear of ill-health.

But although scientific knowledge of disease is constantly increasing, there remain a very large number of disorders, of all grades of severity, for which no real cause or cure is known. For such disorders—and of course they form the bulk of disorders dealt with by psychiatrists—non-scientific medicine has to suffice. I believe that the only useful function of non-scientific medicine lies in the relief of anxiety but, because of the prestige of science, medical procedures which can only relieve anxiety will commonly claim to be scientific. Such a claim, even when manifestly untrue, might be justified on the ground that if a patient thinks them scientific then he will be the more ready to believe in their efficacy. But it is worthwhile to look at present-day medicine to try and see how far its anxiety-relieving functions are appearing in the guise of scientific theory and practice, and also to consider how far some of the conditions now thought to require the attention of doctors have been absorbed into medicine simply because of the decline in prestige of religion and magic.

Anxiety-relieving procedures in medicine

To help us in this inquiry we may note some characteristics of anxiety-relieving procedures in medicine. First, they are not primarily directed towards cure or prevention. Thus the goal of psychoanalysis is often said to be the integration of the personality, and this may or may not be accompanied by relief of the particular symptoms with which the patient presented. This is not necessarily a drawback, for it may lead the patient to resign himself to his symptoms, it may save him from treatments which do more harm than good, and the mere relief of anxiety may—as perhaps in many of the conditions called psychosomatic—strengthen the forces of natural recovery. Secondly, the continued use of anxiety-relieving procedures does not depend upon a demonstration of their therapeutic efficacy. Many books and papers have been written to show that psychotherapy is ineffective but there is no evidence that this has in any way lessened the use or damaged the value of psychotherapy.

A third characteristic of anxiety-relieving procedures is their tendency to take place in an atmosphere of ritual or mystique, or, in the absence of these, to be very costly. Many rituals, those of the operating theatre for example, were of course founded on a proper belief in their need; yet when they are shown to be unnecessary—like the five-minute scrubbing-up period, the face mask and even, some say, the surgeon's gloves—they are still continued, seemingly for their own sake. Ritual and mystique—though not of course cost—are comparatively new in medicine but have always been the stock-in-trade of both religion and magic.

Fourthly, anxiety-relieving procedures are not associated with research into better methods of treatment. True, the techniques of anxiety-relief often change but such changes reflect changes in fashion rather than a response to new assessment of efficacy.

With these characteristics in mind, can we identify anxiety-relieving procedures in medicine of the sort that might at first sight appear to be designed as treatment in the strict sense? I suggest we can. The most obvious is the use of a placebo. The placebo effect depends upon a deliberate deception of a trusting patient, but that can be justified if in fact the patient feels better for it. In prescribing a placebo, the physician is well aware—sometimes uncomfortably aware—of what he is doing, and unless he is capable of being very objective he usually prefers procedures which he can believe are, or at any rate might possibly be, therapeutic in their own right. Hypnosis, and probably acupuncture, are procedures whose immediate usefulness—in terms of anaesthesia, for example—are so obvious that nothing much in the way of theory is thought necessary to justify them. Their main disadvantage of course is that they often do not succeed with sophisticated patients because their efficacy largely depends on uncritical acceptance.

In psychiatry, the most widely accepted form of anxiety-relieving procedure has for many years been psychotherapy. Psychotherapy has the great advantage of being based on theories which have proved capable of satisfying the most intellectual of psychiatrists. It has been observed that the equal success achieved by different schools of psychotherapy betokens a lack of specificity which raises questions about the adequacy of these theories (Eisenberg, 1973). But if the real function of psychotherapy is to relieve anxiety, then the theory by which this is achieved becomes of secondary importance; just as, if we take the real function of religion to be the cure of souls, then we are less inclined to argue that it should be done by one particular religion rather than another.

Anxiety-relieving procedures are of course an essential part of all medical practice but it is reasonable to ask that they should be recognized for what they are and that they should not be allowed to flourish to the extent of endangering health or defrauding the gullible. One could lay down a set of rules. Thus (1) anxiety-relieving procedures should not do more harm than good. This rule is of course particularly applicable when potent drugs are used in effect as placebos. (2) The cost of anxiety-relieving procedures, either to the individual patient or to the state, should not be dispor-portionately high. Individual psychoanalysis is very costly in terms of skilled time. Where the treatment is part of private practice it takes place largely in accordance with the law of supply and demand, but in the setting of a National Health Service its cost-effectiveness must surely be a matter of general concern. Precisely the same may be said of intensive cardiac care units, in so far as these may be catering more for the relief of anxiety than for the cure of disease. (3) We should be ready to make comparative trials of anxiety-relieving procedures. There are problems here, because the anxiety-relieving properties of the waters of Abana and Pharpar are for most people greater than those of the River Jordan. But where therepeutic efficacy is not the test, a comparison on the basis of safety, economy and convenience is still important. (4) Anxiety-relieving procedures should not hinder scientific research. Yet serious attempts to study the efficacy of psychotherapy by con-trolled trials do seem to have met with real if passive resistance (e.g., Candy, 1972). It would of course be of great scientific interest to know whether psychotherapy was therapeutically effective. But even if it could be clearly shown to be ineffective, this would not mean that it should be abandoned. It would simply be revealed as mainly an anxiety-relieving procedure, and in the absence of anything better it would have a proper place in the practice of medicine. Scientific research may be hindered in less immediately obvious ways. During the 1960s, new psychotropic drugs were marketed more quickly than they could properly be assessed, though how far that was part of the scramble for a lucrative market or how far it contained an element of policy is hard to know.

Medicine overloaded

All I have said so far is an attempt to account, in historical terms, for some aspects of the present state of medicine. Because of the decline in prestige of religion and magic and the rise in prestige of medicine, many functions of religion and magic—too many, I suggest—have been loaded on to medicine. This is an inherently unstable state because medicine is unfitted, from its traditions and social structure, to do what religion and magic have done. There are already a number of signs to suggest that some of this overload is beginning to slip away. One of these is what has been called the silent revolution in counselling. An increasing number of non-medical enterprises—Alcoholics Anonymous, the Samaritans, hippy societies, teenage hotlines, encounter groups—concern themselves with problems which over the past 50 years or so had come to be thought of as medical matters. Persons not medically trained—psychologists, social workers, nurses, sociologists—increasingly want to undertake the responsibilities of psychotherapy, which is understandable in a sense, as it looks so easy once one has seen it done. A whole range of patients with problems of the sort that doctors and psychiatrists have recently become accustomed to consider as medical do not want the sort of treatment that doctors conventionally give, but instead want conversation and discussion. Increasingly it seems that patient and doctor have different ideas of what a consultation is for. No doubt it was for these sort of reasons that the Foster report on Scientology (1971) recommended the setting-up of a profession of psychotherapy, open to anyone, medical or lay, who completed a required course of training and accepted an ethical code of conduct.

Another effect of the crowding of anxiety-relief into medicine has been a change in the nature of what is considered illness or disorder. Hysteria has always been of interest to physicians but it is probably only since the time of Thomas Willis, at the end of the seventeenth century, that medicine really took an interest in what we now call nervous disorders; and it is only in the last 50 years that these have been thought to need the attention of a specialist group rather than being merely diagnostic traps for the neurologist. In the last two decades psychiatry has increasingly concerned itself with over-drinking, over-smoking, over- and under-eating, bad driving, marital disharmony, and family problems and minor delinquencies of all kinds. In so far as such problems used to come to the general practitioner he would deal with them by providing such common-sense advice as he, or anyone else, could give; but now they are the subject of research by all respectable academic departments of psychiatry.

The over-burdening of medicine with anxiety-relief may be largely responsible for the strains which have developed between physicians with an interest mainly in the scientific aspects of medicine and those with an interest mainly in its personal aspects. The first sort of doctor is said to see his patient as a case, that is to say, as a biological organism; the second sort of doctor is said to see his patient as a person, that is to say, as a member of a social group. There need be no conflict here so long as both sorts of doctor are aware of the situation.

In new developments, however, especially those in which the community is involved, antagonism is apt to result from an uncertainty of what is what. Thus it is now often believed that scientific

medicine is getting its priorities wrong, with its increasing commitment to the preservation of damaged lives—by organ transplants,
renal dialysis, operations on spina bifida.

One reason for this uncertainty may lie in the conflict which has
developed between the traditional part of medicine—which includes
scientific medicine—and the new medicine which has grown up to
deal with the anxiety-relieving functions taken over from religion
and magic. This conflict has, I suggest, distorted the aims of traditional medicine and led it to concentrate on the application of
science to the relief of sickness, at the expense of its application to
the equally proper and perhaps more important aim of preventing
sickness and maintaining health. It may be that traditional medicine
has avoided concern with community health because the whole
area of social medicine has become confused due to the difficulty of
distinguishing between personal health—the concern of traditional
medicine—and social health—the traditional concern of religion
but now largely taken over by the expanded field of medicine.

Conclusion
I have proposed the thesis that, in Britain over the past three
centuries, the traditional role of religion and magic as relievers of
socially-caused anxiety has declined and that the traditional role of
medicine, as a reliever of anxiety due to ill-health, has been enlarged
to include a responsibility for some socially-caused anxiety. This
process has now proceeded to the extent that medicine as a coherent
system is becoming unstable. The instability reveals itself in ways
which are most clearly evident in psychiatry. The divergence of aim
between those who see medicine primarily in its limited and
traditional role and those who see it primarily in its new enlarged
role has led to the division of psychiatrists into an organic school
and a psychological school. On this view the psychological
psychiatrists concern themselves largely with disorders associated
with socially-induced anxiety. Because the demand for help with
such disorders is exceeding the supply of psychiatrists, non-medical
persons are increasingly acting as 'therapists' and this may lead to
the creation of a new counselling profession not based on medical
training. Such a profession would be reassuming many of the
functions of the priests and astrologers of Jacobean times.

References

Candy, J. and others (1972) A feasibility study for a controlled trial of formal
    psychotherapy. *Psychological Medicine*, 2, 345–62.
Eisenberg, L. (1973) The future of psychiatry. *Lancet, ii*, 1371–5.

Foster, J. G. (1971) *Enquiry into the Practice and Effects of Scientology*. London: HMSO.

Lewis, A. (1953) Health as a social concept, *Brit. J. Sociol.,* **4**, 109–24.

McKeown, T. (1971) The sociological approach to the history of medicine. In *Medical History and Medical Care* (Ed. G. McLaghlan and T. McKeown). London: Oxford University Press.

Thomas, K. (1971) *Religion and the Decline of Magic*. London: Weidenfeld and Nicolson.

AGGRESSION AS A MODE OF COMMUNICATION

P. Slater, I. A. Syed and Sedat Topçu

This is a report on a large but incomplete research project that began just about ten years ago. It started as cross-cultural research in social psychology, proposed by I. A. S. when working with P. S. at the Institute of Psychiatry. He pointed out that the Institute had attracted students from many parts of the Near and Middle East, who had returned to their native countries after taking post-graduate degrees and had since occupied senior academic appointments. There was good hope that some of them would agree to participate in research.

Racial discrimination had become a topic of popular controversy at that time as a result of the influx of immigrants particularly from the West Indies and Pakistan into the UK. Instances of discrimination were frequently reported and inflammatory speeches were being made by demagogues. An attempt to study the subject with scientific impartiality seemed highly desirable.

Konrad Lorenz's book on aggression (1965) led us to entertain the idea that these social phenomena were not wholly due to the special circumstances of the time but were manifestations of tendencies prevalent in the social behaviour of human beings everywhere and throughout history. The exclusion of outsiders is felt to be incumbent on the members of any group who wish to maintain its corporate identity. Similar tendencies are to be found in certain animal species and are important for survival.

If aggressive feelings towards out-groups characterize all human communities, a cross-cultural study should confirm their universal occurrence; and though they may be expressed in different ways, depending on local conditions, they should constitute a personality trait related to other personality traits in a coherent manner.

We chose the title 'Attitudes towards out-groups related to general personality traits' for the research. Psychologists with senior academic appointments in places throughout the Near and Middle East were to be asked whether such aggressive feelings were observable in the communities where they worked, and if so, whether they would construct a 'prejudice scale' for inclusion in the cross-cultural research, using phrases current in their community for indicating hostile feelings towards the groups regarded locally as out-groups.

The scale would consist of typical statements for expressing or repudiating feelings of hostility. They would be combined in a randomized order with statements for measuring six other personality traits, taken from questionnaires validated in previous researches, to make up a general 'inventory of social attitudes'. Subjects would be asked to respond by indicating agreement or disagreement with them on a five-point scale. A battery of five other tests would also be given, including Group Test 70/1, a non-verbal intelligence test published by the National Institute of Industrial Psychology.

To avoid political embarrassment the researches were to be independent of each other in certain important respects though all designed on a common plan. The prejudice scales were to be devised specially for each research, and were not to include any reference to foreigners; the rest of the test material was to be the same. Each participant was to be responsible for collecting the data in his own district; the data from each district were then to be analysed by P. S. separately, though with the same mathematical methods; and each participant would receive the results from his own data and be personally responsible for their interpretation.

Preliminary enquiries were addressed to suitable people in the areas concerned, and favourable replies were received. An application for a year's research grant to make a preliminary survey of the possibilities was submitted to the Social Science Research Council, and a grant was received with effect from spring 1968.

Work began with collecting data from an English sample, and meanwhile arrangements were made to visit potential participants. Plans were interrupted by the six-days war between Israel and Egypt and Syria. But after some delays and rerouting, visits were paid to Egypt, Iran, Iraq, Israel, Jordan, the Lebanon, Turkey, five centres in India, three in West Pakistan and two in East Pakistan (now Bangladesh). Contacts were also made with Syria and the Sudan.

No-one was found to be in any doubt that feelings of hostility to local out-groups were prevalent in their communities. Even in the heart of India, where foreign countries seem almost as remote as the moon, hostile feelings were rife between Hindus, Sikhs, Moslems and other smaller cultural groups. We received assurances of participation everywhere except in the Lebanon, where it was refused on the grounds that the situation there was so tense that enquiries into hostile feelings between different groups might precipitate public disorder. It was difficult to believe this could be so in the atmosphere of peace and prosperity prevalent then, but subsequent events have justified the fears of the authorities.

We returned feeling that we had made all the necessary arrangements for a cross-cultural research covering a very wide area. But P.S. had also returned with a tropical sprue which made him very ill and weak for several months. Whether because of this or because of the precariousness of the political situation, or for any other reason, the SSRC refused to support the project any further. However, it was not completely abandoned.

Data were collected by Professor S. Jalota in Raipur, India, by Dr Y. Rim in Israel, and by Sedat Topçu under the direction of Professor F. K. Gökay in Turkey. Later Sedat Topçu came to England to study for a Ph.D. degree. Besides examining the data from the large-scale investigations in Turkey, Israel and England, he added a fresh dimension to the scope of the research by making detailed case-studies of 75 psychiatric inpatients at Netherne Hospital: 30 with records of overt violence, 15 with records of suicidal attempts, and a control group of 30 patients with no such records. It is because of his perseverance and initiative that useful results have been extracted from both investigations: the cross-cultural study and his own original research work. The results are reported in his Ph.D. thesis 'Psychological concomitants of aggressive feelings and behaviour' (1976).

The results from the cross-cultural survey confirmed Lorenz's theory substantially. The most convincing evidence was the unanimity of expert opinion in all the countries we contacted, that aggressive feelings towards minority groups in their communities were strong, widespread and easy to observe. Moreover the detailed analyses of the data from England, Israel and Turkey showed similar associations between the local scales of prejudice and the reference scales for other psychological variables. For example, in all three countries prejudice was found positively associated with authoritarianism, conservatism, intolerance of ambiguity, and social distance towards out-groups. The results from Raipur were inconclusive because although the prejudice scale proved internally consistent the other attitude scales did not.

The findings brought to special attention here concern the relation between intelligence and aggression. The results from the cross-cultural studies show no association whatever between scores on the prejudice scales and scores on the non-verbal intelligence tests. The correlations are:

−.052 in the English sample of 185 cases
−.035 in the Israeli sample of 192 cases
.022 in the Turkish sample of 218 cases

In short there is no evidence of any connection between aggressive *feelings* and intelligence.

Topçu's results from Netherne Hospital concerning intelligence are interestingly different. The patients were given both a verbal and a nonverbal test (the Mill Hill Vocabulary Test and the Progressive Matrices Test). The average score of the patients with records of acts of violence was lower than the average of the control group on both tests; and a covariance analysis shows that the mean score of the aggressive patients on the verbal test was significantly lower than expected, taking the difference in their mean scores on the non-verbal test into account. The details are reported in Topçu's thesis.

From this evidence it appears important to distinguish between aggressive feelings and aggressive behaviour. People are equally prone to aggressive feelings whatever the level of their intelligence but those who express their feelings by action have a lower level on the average and are differentially less able to put their feelings into words.

Lorenz's theory of aggression is relevant to these findings also. According to him aggressive behaviour towards others of their own kind occurs in certain animal species, although not all, and is generally valuable to the survival of the species. It arises usually in disputes over territory or mastery of herds of females, and the consequences are generally beneficial, leading to more even distribution of feeding-grounds or the propagation of the species by the most potent males.

Fighting between animals, he adds, takes the form of single combat at close quarters using the weapons provided by nature: claws, hooves, horns, jaws, etc. It seldom results in death; it is terminated by a gesture of submission by one of the combatants which inhibits further aggressive behaviour by the acknowledged victor.

In man, however, historical events have produced a pathological over-development of aggressiveness. Weapons have been introduced into combat and have become steadily more lethal and effective at greater distances. Individual gestures of submission have lost their power to elicit any immediate response. Campaigns are planned long in advance. The individual soldier, acting under orders, is exonerated from all feelings of guilt, the victor is acclaimed as a hero and the successful commander is loaded with honour and glory.

According to this theory the association we have found between intelligence and aggressiveness can be explained by supposing that more intelligent people, though no less prone to aggressive feelings than others, are more inclined to be influenced by inhibitory processes. The common observation that over-indulgence in alcohol is liable to lead to aggressive behaviour may also be explained in the same way: aggressive feelings may not be increased—they are presumably on tap at all times—but inhibitory processes are weakened and consequently slighter provocation is sufficient to convert the feelings into behaviour.

There are plenty of other theories about aggression, perhaps the most influential being the frustration—aggression hypothesis advanced by Dollar *et al.* in 1939. It avoids Lorenz's assumption that aggression is instinctive and offers a behaviouristic explanation that when drives directed towards other goals are obstructed they are liable to be diverted into aggressive behaviour. This theory does not appear to fit the results of the researches reported here but it may account for some other manifestations of aggression and thus help to explain how widespread aggressive behaviour is. All kinds of drives may reinforce it. And what happens when aggression itself is frustrated? According to the main doctrine of behaviourism conditioned responses are gradually extinguished when they are not reinforced with any reward. According to the logic of the frustration–aggression theory, however, when a drive which has become aggressive is unrewarded it is liable to be reinforced further or else diverted into another outlet. This would account for the kind of aggressive behaviour typified as 'kicking the cat'.

We see no reason to reject one theory of aggression because a different one helps to explain the phenomena. The effects of aggression are so widespread and often so catastrophic that any theory that can explain a few of them deserves careful consideration, and any further theory that can extend our understanding is to be welcomed.

In the theories discussed so far aggression has not been examined sufficiently carefully in our opinion as an interpersonal relationship. It is not just an attitude of mind or a type of behaviour but an approach of one person to another, generally with the intention of imposing his will on the other. In this respect it is a substitute for conversation and persuasion: in other words an alternative mode of communication. In the discussion which follows we are expressing opinions which go beyond the evidence but which have been considered in the light of it and agreed.

When aggression is viewed as a mode of communication the behaviour of the defendant comes into consideration as well as that of the aggressor. Scene: a crowded place.

'Excuse me', says aggressor, 'would you mind letting me get past?'

Defendant remains with back turned, makes no movement and says nothing.
Aggressor taps him on the shoulder and repeats, rather more loudly, 'Let me past, please!'
Defendant turns round, stares him blankly in the face and makes no effort to let him go by.
'Come on, get out of my way, you bastard!', says aggressor giving him a hearty shove.
Defendant retaliates. Punch-up starts. Bystanders join in.

Thus one mode of communication becomes translated into another, aggression being the mode used when others fail.

Aggressive action has served as a means of communication between persons in power and their subordinates since the dawn of history. Rules are made and disobedience is punished. Punishments come in all shapes and sizes: parents punish their children 'to teach them a lesson'. Sentences are pronounced in courts of law on one offender to serve as a warning to others not to copy his behaviour. The offender is not considered entitled to any reply to this kind of communication.

Yet legal systems are not invariably in the best interests of the governed. In history, as distinct from political theory, the governments of most states have been established by foreigners, who have brought the local inhabitants under their domination by conquest and introduced legal systems for maintaining themselves in power. In course of time customs change, rulers and ruled are intermingled and tend to become united, democratic processes modify the legal system to remove injustices and make it conform more closely to what the population considers is right.

Or else, communication addressed by the oppressed to the oppressors is liable to take increasingly aggressive forms: passive resistance, non-violent non-cooperation, sabotage, insurrection, revolution. The findings of the Netherne experiment are relevant to this process of transition towards progressively more violent modes of communication. It is to be expected that some of the members of any minority group with a grievance will be more intelligent and articulate than others. The earliest expressions of grievance are likely to come from them. If these are ignored the members expressing them will become discredited, more aggressive modes of communication will be adopted and the leadership will pass to the less intelligent and articulate members, who are readier to resort to violence. Opportunities for quiet reasonable resolution of disagreements will have been lost.

A government which intends to be just should be ready to receive communications promptly from anybody with a reasonable complaint. It needs a receptor system to match its effector system. In terms of Shakespeare's favourite analogy between the body politic and the human body the two systems should act as coordinated parts of the central nervous system. When taking a hot bath we test the heat of the water from the hot-water tap with our finger-tips, and if it is too hot we turn the cold tap as well. We adjust the temperature with repeated testing as the bath fills and make a final test with one foot before entering. The whole operation proceeds smoothly because the receptor system and the motor system are acting in conjunction. A government without an efficient receptor system, if it decides that the body politic needs a hot bath, may plunge it completely into water that is actually boiling hot or icy cold.

Any large-scale social engineering, however well-intentioned and likely to be beneficial in the long run, is liable to impose stress and hardship on some sections of the community, if only temporarily. Their grievances may be expressed in many ways: by surreptitious evasive action, public petitions or demonstrations, or eventually by overt aggressive behaviour. When this occurs it may not necessarily be directed at the original source of the grievance, but may attack any part of the body politic that is exposed and sensitive. The message may not have much chance of getting through when it is transmitted in such ways. The person who delivers it may not be able to explain it and the one who receives it may not be the one for whom it is intended. The aggressive action may seem completely irrational, for though it may speak louder than words it may drown sense in noise.

If no attempt is made to decipher it and reply to it reasonably, the reply actually sent may be no less aggressive and irrational though it may be dictated by policy or law. A kind of conversation ensues which rapidly becomes more heated, barbaric and unintelligible. People with no idea what it is all about may interrupt and confuse the issue. The message becomes continually more indecipherable.

Good government, especially if it intends to introduce social changes, needs a receptor system rapidly responsive to grievances and a smooth efficient procedure for attending to them and mitigating them before they become aggravated. As the Chinese philosopher Lao Tzu once said (Waley, 1934):

In the governance of empire everything difficult must be dealt with while it is still easy.

Everything great must be dealt with while it is still small.

Therefore the sage never has to deal with the great, and so achieves greatness.

References

Dollar, J., Miller, N., Doob, L., Mowrer, O. H. & Sears, R. R. (1939) *Frustration and Aggression*. New Haven: Yale University Press.

Lorenz, K. (1956) *On Aggression*. London: Methuen.

Topçu, S. (1976) *Psychological concomitants of aggressive feelings and behaviour*. Thesis for Ph. D. degree, University of London.

Waley, A. (1934) *The way and its power. A study of the Tao Te Ching and its place in Chinese thought*. London: George Allen and Unwin.

EPILEPSY

EXPERIMENTAL EPILEPSY IN MONKEYS

G. Ettlinger

Introduction

Historical

The field of investigation now called neuropsychology developed in Great Britain with the benevolent encouragement of Eliot Slater. His department at the National Hospital accepted administrative responsibility for a small group of neuropsychologists as long ago as the late 1940s. This team was led by Oliver Zangwill and included John McFie and Malcolm Piercy. At that time their chief interest lay in the effects of restricted brain lesions on complex human behaviour: the association between the site of the cortical lesion and selective intellectual defects; the relationship between disease of left or right parietal cortex and defective spatial performance; and cerebral dominance, especially in sinistrals. Such work still continues today in the Department of Psychological Medicine at the National Hospital.

In 1957 British neuropsychology took a new direction: the systematic behavioural study of monkeys subjected to experimental neurosurgical procedures. In the hands of Karl Lashley, Heinrich Klüver and many others, such work had long prospered in the USA. It had also thrived for shorter periods in the UK, for example, in the laboratories of David Ferrier, Sir Edward Schäfer (=Sharpey-Schäfer), Victor Horsley, Sir Charles Sherrington and Paul Glees. Owing to the interests of Oliver Zangwill, similar work began in the Psychological Laboratory at Cambridge in 1957 where it still flourishes today. It was also started at the National Hospital later in the same year with the support of Arnold Carmichael, John Bates and of course Eliot Slater. Monkey behaviour research has spread widely throughout the UK since that time, and has found a place also in departments of anatomy, and of physiology.

Even in the setting of a large neurological hospital with its clinical orientation, it soon became evident that the drawbacks of primate

147

behaviour research—the risks of over-ready extrapolation to man and the limited behavioural repertoire of monkeys—were largely counterbalanced by the greater control afforded to the investigator: control over the previous behavioural and neurological histories of the subjects; over the precise limits and nature of the imposed brain lesion; over the behavioural measures and over the ultimate verification of the neurosurgical procedures. Given Eliot Slater's observations on the association between temporal lobe epilepsy and psychosis, and given the interest of George Dawson, my Departmental Head at the Institute of Psychiatry after 1962, in the physiological processes underlying epilepsy, it seems natural in retrospect that a proportion of my work should have become directed toward experimental epilepsy.

Scientific

Three claims in particular attracted my attention. First, Stamm and his associates (Stamm and Pribram, 1960; Stamm and Pribram, 1961) reported findings which to them suggested that an epileptogenic or discharging lesion influences the monkey's behaviour in a qualitatively different way from a surgical ablation of the comparable cortical region. I was not aware of any comparable observations in man. Did the findings then represent a difference in brain organization between man and monkey? Or were there important differences in methodology?

Secondly, Ward and his colleagues (Calvin, Sypert and Ward, 1968; Ward, 1969) claimed to have shown that single cells in an experimental cortical discharging focus have a characteristic pattern of firing. (Since then Calvin, Ojemann and Ward, 1973, have reported a similar pattern of discharge of 'epileptic' nurones in man). However, they had studied only primary foci, induced in animals by the injection of a chemical agent into the cortex. Was the pattern of discharge truly representative of all 'epileptic' neurones, including those in secondary foci which occur in cortex not directly subjected to experimental procedures?

Third, Westrum *et al* (1965) and Ward (1969) described structural changes in the neurones of the monkey's epileptogenic focus. For example, the Golgi stain revealed malformation of the apical dendrites together with loss of dendritic spines. However, again the evidence for this important claim derived at that time from neurones in the experimental primary focus (apart from a reference by Scheibel and Scheibel, 1968, to their then unpublished but now published (1974) observations of similar structural changes in man). The objection could be raised that the changes in the primary experimental focus were, perhaps, an effect of the chemical agent used to induce abnormal discharges in the monkey and not an effect of the abnormal discharges. Such objections have been countered by the authors who found structural alterations only in foci of monkeys not treated by anticonvulsant drugs. However, it remained remotely possible that the anticonvulsants had interacted with the chemical epileptogenic agent so as to prevent this agent from producing the structural changes. Would the structural changes also be observed in secondary foci which have never been treated chemically but originate as a consequence of the discharging activity of the primary focus?

To me it seemed that each of these problems raised issues of major importance. Their resolution could, however, be tackled only as the relevant technologies were mastered. So first, we set about producing primary and secondary foci reliably. The epileptogenic effects of aluminium hydroxide, cortical freezing, metallic cobalt, penicillin, tungstic acid gel and cerebromeningeal scars were studied (in collaboration with G. Dawson and H. B. Morton). Once the first was selected as most suitable for producing long-lasting primary discharges, further work (in collaboration with Miss A. Moffett, M. V. Driver, Mrs D. Gautrin and G. Fenton) indicated the necessary conditions for the reliable development of secondary foci. At this stage we were ready to investigate the comparative effects of discharging lesions and cortical removals on the complex behaviour of the monkey (see section A1).

The same techniques also enabled us to seek an answer to another question, posed by Geschwind (1965): can prolonged epileptiform discharges 'open up' or 'make available' brain pathways not normally available for the mediation of complex behaviour? Geschwind supposed that the absence of behavioural impairment in some cases of human brain bisection was due to their longstanding epileptic discharges. These discharges might, he supposed, have opened up interhemispheric pathways below the level of the diencephalon, so that in these (but not in more acutely) epileptic patients the two cerebral hemispheres were interconnected even after neocortical commissure section. Fortunately for us, Mr J. J. Maccabe had for several years been sectioning the forebrain commissures in monkeys required for other work unrelated to epilepsy. The behavioural aspects of this study are described in Section A2, and some totally unexpected electrical findings consequent upon this experiment in Section B1.

A totally different technology was required for recording from single cells in the epileptic focus. The main requirements were that: (1) the animal be undrugged and unanaesthetized; (2) recordings be taken without bolting the head to a rigid frame (as was the practice in USA at that time); (3) electrodes be passed to temporal cortex on the ventral surface of the brain, without the electrode breaking as it passed through cortex *outwards* (i.e. dorso-ventrally) towards the floor of the skull; (4) provision be made for recording from two or three cells concurrently. This technology was developed during three years in collaboration with J. D. Cooper, F. H. Goldsmith, H. B. Morton, B. Moss and S. Ackley. We were then able to record with up to three microelectrodes from temporal cortical neurones in the undrugged and only lightly restrained monkey for periods of three or more hours. Much of the credit for the development of the final system of recording belongs to Mrs D. Gautrin, my scientific colleague at that time. Miss B. Frost, and later Miss V. Nie, collaborated in the subsequent collection of data as described in Section B2.

Thanks to the help of G. S. Garcha, the Golgi technique of neural staining is now available to us and has been applied to primary and secondary foci by Mrs M. B. Lowrie. This work is further discussed in Section C1.

Experiments
A1 Differential behavioural effects of discharges and ablations?
Stamm and his associates (1960, 1961) claimed that epileptogenic lesions in the monkey impair the learning of new tasks but do not impair the retention (or relearning) of tasks first mastered before the onset of the discharges. It is widely accepted that cortical removals in the monkey impair not only new learning but also retention of previously learnt tasks. The evidence from man is inconclusive, but suggests (as does certain evidence from animal experiments) that impaired cognitive performance is more likely to be associated with epilepsy than with cortical destruction (Blakemore *et al*, 1966).

One way of resolving the discrepant findings was to alter the training procedures used by Stamm and his colleagues for the assessment of retention in monkeys made epileptic: during the months of waiting for the discharges to appear, these animals (but not the animals with cortical ablations) had been repeatedly retrained—although it was already known that such repeated training (also termed 'overtraining') eliminated retention defects in animals having cortical ablations. Therefore, in an investigation reported by Moffett *et al* (1970) the basic procedures of Stamm and Warren (1961) were adapted so that all of the monkeys were retrained on previously learnt tasks only once, namely after the onset of the discharges in the EEGs of the experimental animals. No differential effects on learning and retention were then found within the group of animals with discharging lesions. Instead, suggestions emerged that cortical destruction was of greater relevance for behavioural defect than the abnormal electrical discharges. This view received confirmation from the subsequent work of Gautrin *et al* (1971) and of Nie *et al* (1973): in the monkey the discharging lesions resulting from the application of aluminium hydroxide seemed to influence behaviour by virtue of the associated cortical destruction consequent upon the application of the epileptogenic agent to the pial surface and not by virtue of the undoubted electrical discharges also produced by the agent.

These experiments on the monkey taken together with the directly relevant clinical study of Blakemore *et al* (1966) suggest: (i) in the monkey discharges do not influence behaviour in a qualitatively different way from removals of cortex as had been repeatedly claimed by others; (ii) in the monkey impaired performance consequent to the application of aluminium hydroxide does not result from the electrical abnormalities, as had been claimed by others, but from destruction of cortex by the chemical agent; (iii) the closer association in man of cognitive impairment with discharges than with neuropathological damage has yet to be documented in monkeys—but the clinical and animal investigations have differed in various ways (e.g. the age of the subjects at the time of the onset of the discharges and the kind of behaviour investigated).

A2 Can discharges open up new pathways?
Geschwind (1965) supposed that long-standing epileptic discharges open up interhemispheric pathways not normally accessible for the mediation of complex behaviour. This would explain: (a) the good performance (on many tasks of interhemispheric integration) after commissure section by certain patients with epilepsy presumed to be consequent upon birth injuries; and (b) the poor performance after similar surgery on the same tasks by patients with epilepsy consequent upon trauma later in life. However, no direct evidence exists for or against Geschwind's view. Moreover, the discrepant findings in cases of brain bisections have been accounted for in other ways: by Gazzaniga and Sperry (1967) as due to greater cortical destruction in the cases of head injury; by the present author (at a lecture in 1969) as due to more efficient post-surgical learning in the cases without head injury.

With J. J. Maccabe, Miss V. Nie and M. Hunter we prepared eight monkeys in 1971: four with total section of the corpus callosum, massa intermedia and anterior and posterior commissures and also left parieto-occipital epileptogenic lesions; and four control animals (with similar lesions except that either 5–8 mm of corpus callosum were intentionally spared or a parieto-occipital ablation was performed instead of applying the epileptogenic agent). The intention was to follow for a year the discharges in these animals with monthly EEG recordings and to correlate the amount of transfer of tactile information between the hands with either the amount of discharging activity or with the surgical status.

In the event, we had a severe outbreak of TB in the monkey colony during 1971 and 1972, which necessitated the curtailment of the work. Mr. M. Hunter was able to assess tactile transfer in only one experimental and one control animal. He found better than expected performance in the experimental animal on five out of six tactile tasks (see Hunter, Maccabe and Ettlinger, 1976).

Histological examination subsequently indicated total commissure section in the experimental animal. (Attempts to replicate this finding in three further monkeys failed when they developed sensory defect in the hand contralateral to the chronic primary discharges, M. B. Lowrie and G. Ettlinger, unpublished.) This preliminary finding therefore supports Geschwind's proposal, and can be explained by recalling that there are two routes of ipsilateral somato-sensory projection (cf Innocenti *et al,* 1973). In the former, the inflow passes to the contralateral sensory cortex and then through callosal fibres to the ipsilateral sensory area; in the latter there is a direct, uncrossed path to the ipsilateral cortex. This latter projection is not functional in the split-brain monkey which fails to show tactile transfer, but it might be activated by abnormal discharges from parietal cortex in an 'epileptic' monkey if the discharges interfere predominantly with the crossed projection pathway.

B1 How do discharges spread to the second hemisphere after commissure section?

As part of the behavioural experiment already described in Section A2, monkeys with total division of all forebrain commissures and of the massa intermedia were given at the same operation a unilateral parieto-occipital epileptogenic implant. To our surprise all four monkeys showed evidence of independent secondary mirror foci (i.e. discharges from the second hemisphere that were unrelated in time to primary discharges) as described by Nie *et al* (1974). The time-course of the development of the independent mirror foci was variable but the EEG evidence was quite convincing (see Figure 1). Nevertheless, Mrs M. B. Lowrie, Mr J. J. Maccabe and I have prepared similar animals. In four the primary foci were ablated, in three the secondary foci. Primary and transmitted secondary discharges ceased after primary ablations but were unaffected by removals of the secondary cortex; independent secondary discharges persisted after removals of the primary focus but were abolished by secondary ablations (Lowrie *et al,* 1978).

The way in which the secondary foci were able to develop is of particular interest here. Nie *et al* (1974) discussed certain possible

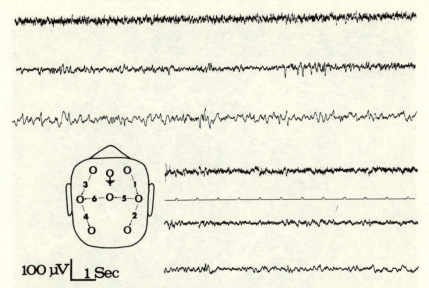

Fig. 1. EEG tracing from monkey David at five months after commissure section and implantation of aluminium hydroxide on the left parietal cortex. HF cut 15 per cent at 50 Hz; TC=0.03 sec. There is a clear burst of independent discharges from the right (secondary) hemisphere.

factors. They preferred a process of neural transmission along inter-hemispheric connections (e.g. in the hypothalamus or reticular formation) that had not been divided surgically. However, since their report was written some new evidence and ideas have emerged, many of which are discussed by Lowrie *et al* (1978).

Dr J. Wilden and I have studied the transmission of discharges from a unilateral parieto-occipital penicillin focus in two monkeys with total neocortical commissure section and in two control animals without prior neurosurgical intervention (unpublished observations). These animals did not develop independent foci but all four showed clear and unambiguous secondary events, transmitted from the primary hemisphere (see Figure 2a). Although after a period of 28 hours a proportion of secondary events tended to have latencies of about 10 msec, much earlier during the record-ings all secondary events were of zero or near zero msec latency (see Figure 2b). The interpretation of these recent findings is still unclear. Nevertheless, they may throw light on the development of the secondary focus in commissure sectioned animals. Also, Ettlinger and Lowrie (1976) have proposed an immunological factor in epilepsy, an idea which is elaborated below in the Discussion. In any case, it could be argued that commissure section may be an inappropriate therapeutic procedure for existing bilateral epilepsy in man if such surgery does not prevent the spread to the second hemisphere of unilateral epilepsy in the monkey.

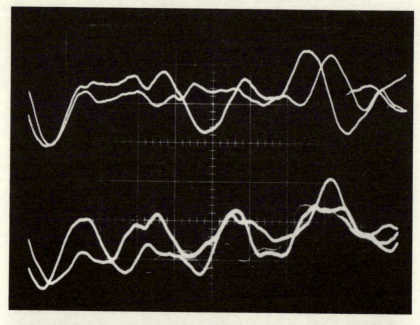

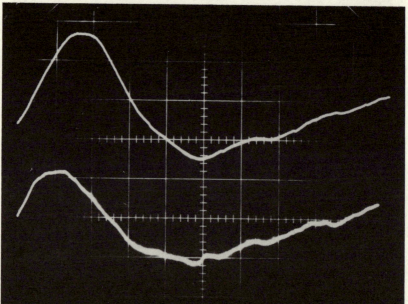

Fig. 2. (a) Primary (lower trace) and secondary (upper trace) discharges in monkey Dostojevsky at 5 hrs after application of penicillin to the left (primary) parieto-occipital cortex. Time is 20 msec/div. HF cut at 50 Hz; TC=0.03 sec. (b) The same but at 28 hrs after surgery. Time is 10 msec/div. The epileptogenic focus was produced at 17 months after section of the corpus callosum, massa intermedia, anterior and posterior commissures; and at 14 months after division of the cerebellum. From unpublished observations by J. Wilden and G. Ettlinger.

B2 What are the first changes in the pattern of neuronal discharge during the development of the secondary focus?

In the monkey, the ventral temporal cortex mediates visual discrimination performance. Since we ultimately wished to study the neuronal basis of learnt performance (see Ridley and Ettlinger, 1973; Ridley *et al,* 1977) and the interaction of epileptic discharges with learnt performance we decided in 1968 to develop a method of recording from single cells in this particular cortical region. The method has been described elsewhere by Cooper *et al* (1972) and by Cooper and Hewett (1975). It enables us to record on magnetic tape the electrical potentials from several cells concurrently. One cell might be situated in the primary focus, the other in a corresponding region of the contralateral hemisphere. At the same time we record the standard scalp EEG on paper. Certain selected EEG or ECoG channels are also recorded on magnetic tape. This permits the pattern of cell activity to be correlated with the standard scalp EEG or with the 'local' ECoG, the slow mass cortical activity at the site of the microelectrode.

Our method of producing primary foci in ventral temporal cortex has been fully described elsewhere by Gautrin *et al* (1971) and by Nie *et al* (1973). Of importance is that we apply the chemical agent to the pial surface in celluloid caps, whereas Ward and his colleagues inject it intra-cortically. (We too have tried the method of injection: with our injections the aluminium hydroxide spread more widely and produced EEG changes that were less focal and specific.) It is also important that secondary transmitted or independent foci develop in the majority of our animals (Nie *et al*, 1973) whereas this is not the case in Ward's laboratory (Harris, 1972). The discrepancy could result from differences in the application of the chemical agent or in the site of the application—motor cortex is the site in Ward's laboratory, whereas we use ventral temporal (or parieto-occipital) cortex. Nie and Ettlinger (1974) and Lowrie *et al* (1978) have shown that our secondary independent temporal and parietal foci (as judged by EEG asynchronies) can survive, although with a somewhat diminished activity, the widespread ablation of the primary focus.

The analysis of our unit recordings in primary and secondary foci is still incomplete. After two years of analysis by photography, the difficulties of triggering reliably from epileptic events indicated the advantages of further analysis by computer. This has been undertaken by Dr O. Holmes. However, some preliminary findings (all based only on photography) may be presented: (1) neither in the primary nor in the secondary focus have we seen patterns of discharge ('long first interval bursts') which have been described by Calvin *et al* (1968) as characteristic of neuronal discharges in epileptic foci; (ii) relatively few cells discharge in a way that is obviously related to EEG or ECoG activity; (iii) when cells are related to either EEG or ECoG activity there is a preponderance of inhibition, i.e. decrease in rate of discharge from the resting rate; (iv) cells in the secondary focus can be time-locked to either ictal or interictal EEG or ECoG events in the primary hemisphere, usually showing a reduced rate of discharge for about 200msec; (v) time-locking of secondary cells to primary ictal events has been seen as early as eight weeks after application of the epileptogenic agent to the primary hemisphere (see Figure 3).

Further discussion of these findings must await detailed publication of the results (Holmes, Ettlinger and Nie, in preparation). However, it is evident that work of this kind on the secondary focus has certain advantages: this focus develops as a result of or in association with, neural discharges from the primary focus but in cortex free from direct experimental intervention, so that it should serve as a generic model of the epileptic process. (In contrast, study

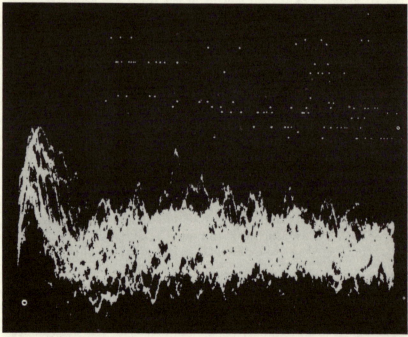

Figure 3. Cell 27571R4 from monkey Ermine at eight weeks after left temporal epileptogenic implant with aluminium hydroxide. The rows of dots are successive discharges of the cell (one dot indicates one action potential) over periods of 500 msec triggered by the primary EEG discharges in the superimposed lower traces. The cell was situated in the secondary hemisphere; the EEG is derived from the temporal to occipital leads of the primary hemisphere and forms part of a seizure. From unpublished observations by G. Ettlinger and V. Nie.

of the primary focus is beset by difficulties of interpretation because any findings could be specific to the particular mode of primary epileptogenesis.)

C1 Are there structural alterations of the neurones in the epileptic focus?
We, like others, have looked for neuronal changes in the foci of our animals, and with Nissl stain have found none in the secondary focus. Now Mrs M. B. Lowrie has made Golgi preparations but her findings are not yet available. Emphasis will again fall on secondary foci as uncontaminated by experimental procedures, but she will also examine primary foci.

This kind of work has clear implication for the understanding of the epileptic process. Controversy persists as to whether neurones are in any way abnormal or whether only the pattern of discharge of normal neurones is disordered.

Discussion
In the clinic epilepsy has many manifestations. Even within one patient it is variable and fluctuating. The most appropriate experimental models in animals will replicate this variability. This is what enhances the difficulties of research on epilepsy—there are weeks or months of waiting for the phenomenon to be investigated to appear, and then it is fluctuating. (One recourse is to activate the epileptic process—but this procedure introduces difficulties of interpretation, i.e. whether a finding is related to epilepsy or to the procedure used to activate it.)

Despite these difficulties there has in recent years been considerable progress in understanding the features of the epileptic process. Ward and his colleagues have led the way with a multi-disciplinary approach—clinical, electrophysiological, histological and biochemical. Their work has served as a source of encouragement to others investigating epilepsy—by indicating lines of research that are likely to be fruitful, and by their persistence in not being deflected into other branches of neurobiology by the difficulties of this field.

Most recently there have been proposals by Ettlinger and Lowrie (1976) and by Cazzullo *et al* (1976) that certain kinds of epileptic discharge may originate as an auto-immune response to antigens released by a variety of kinds of tissue destruction. Antibodies to such antigens may then occupy receptor sites, preventing synaptic transmission in presumably inhibitory systems. The direct evidence for such views remains to be gathered (but see Cazzullo *et al*, 1976). Some indirect evidence is presented in Table 1. In 20 of 55 monkeys secondary events anteceded (5) or were recorded in the same monthly EEG (15) as primary events; in 35 monkeys primary events occurred first (but 21 of these animals showed no independent secondary discharges). This pattern of onset of primary and secondary discharges could hardly be expected if the secondary discharges are a consequence of neural bombardment from an earlier primary focus. Since secondary foci are generally in corresponding cortical areas regional specificity of transmitter agents would support an immunological process. At the moment there exists evidence only for regional specificity of antibodies (Mihailović and Čupić, 1971).

In this country there has been more clinical than basic work on epilepsy, even though treatment by anticonvulsants is still empirical.

TABLE I

Incidence of monkeys with primary or secondary events occurring either first in time or exclusively

	Primary first (no secondary independent discharges)	Secondary first (no primary discharges)	Both together (primary and secondary independent)
Gautrin *et al.* (1971)	3, 5, 6, 8 1*, 2*, 3*, 4*, 5*, 7*	—	2, 7, 10
In 4 animals, i.e. 1, 4, 9 & 6* impossible to ascertain			
Nie *et al.* (1973)	3, 4, 7, 9, 10, 11 1*	1	2, 5, 6, 8
In 4 animals, i.e. 12–15 impossible to ascertain			
Nie & Ettlinger (unpublished) 4 animals not re-counted. In 1 animal impossible to ascertain	5, 8, 10		1, 2, 4, 6, 7, 9
Nie *et al.* (1974)	1, 2, 3		4
Lowrie *et al.* (1978)	3, 4, 5, 6, 8, 11, 12, 13, 14, 15, 16*, 17	2, 7, 9, 10	1
Totals	35	5	15

Numbers in table refer to designations of individual monkeys used in presenting the observations; but totals are arithmetical sums of columns.

*Indicates animals published but shown to have no secondary events of any kind.

Nonetheless, the time seems opportune to take another look at the basic problems. The purpose of this brief review has been to recapitulate Eliot Slater's influence on experimental as well as clinical neuropsychology; and to suggest that there exists at the present time the need for further investigations of many kinds into the underlying mechanisms of the epileptic process.

Summary
The influence of Eliot Slater on the development of neuropsychology in Britain is traced. His example was partly instrumental in the launching of a programme of research work on the epileptic process.

A series of experiments on the behavioural and electrophysiological manifestations of experimental epilepsy in the monkey is briefly recounted. Certain of the findings are new; others cast doubt upon claims to be found in the literature. It is concluded that the time seems ripe for a variety of further experimental studies in this area.

Acknowledgements
I am grateful to my colleagues who have been associated with me in this work; to Professor G. D. Dawson and the late Dr E. A. Carmichael who guided us at various stages; to the MRC who have provided financial support for very many years; and to the Wellcome Trust for supporting the work on unit recording in 1972–1975.

References
Blakemore, C. B., Ettlinger, G. & Falconer, M. A. (1966) Cognitive abilities in relation to frequency of seizures and neuropathology of the temporal lobes in man. *J. Neurol. Neurosurg. Psychiat.*, 29, 268–72.

Calvin, W. H., Sypert, G. W. & Ward, A. A. (1968) Structured timing patterns within bursts from epileptic neurons in undrugged monkey cortex. *Exp. Neurol.* 21, 535–49.

Calvin, W. H., Ojemann, G. A. & Ward, A. A. (1973) Human cortical neurons in epileptogenic foci: comparison of inter-ictal firing patterns to those of "epileptic" neurons in animals. *Electroenceph. Clin. Neurophysiol.*, 34, 337–51.

Cazzullo, C. L., Altamura, A. L., Canger, R. & Penati, G. (1976) Cobalt-induced epilepsy in cats pharmacologically immunodepressed. *Arzneim.-Forsch*, 26, 1387–93.

Cooper, J. D., Ettlinger, G. & Goldsmith, F. H. (1972) A method of recording unit activity from ventral temporal cortex in the undrugged and lightly restrained monkey. *J. Physiol*, 222, 133–4P.

Cooper, J. D. & Hewett, T. D. (1975) Remote control system for very small microelectrode advancers. *J. Physiol.*, 237, 13–15P.

Ettlinger, G. & Lowrie, M. B. (1976) An immunological factor in epilepsy. *Lancet, i*, 1386.

Gazzaniga, M. S. & Sperry, R. W. (1967) Language after section of the cerebral commissures. *Brain*, 90, 131—48.

Gautrin, D., Fenton, G. & Ettlinger, G. (1971) Aluminium hydroxide implants on the inferotemporal cortex of the monkey: their mode of influencing visual discrimination performance. *Exper. Neurol.*, 33, 459–74.

Geschwind, N. (1965) In *Functions of the Corpus Callosum* (ed. E. G. Ettlinger) Ciba Found. Study Group No 20. J. & A. Churchill.

Harris, A. B. (1972) Degeneration in experimental epileptic foci. *Arch. Neurol. Chicago*, 26, 434–49.

Hunter, M., Maccabe, J. J. & Ettlinger, G. (1976) Transfer of training between the hands in a split-brain monkey with chronic parietal discharges. *Cortex*, 12, 27–30.

Innocenti, G. M., Manzoni, T. & Spidalieri, G. (1973) Relevance of the callosal transfer in defining the peripheral reactivity of somesthetic cortical neurones. *Arch. Ital. Biol.*, 111, 187–221.

Lowrie, M. B., Maccabe, J. J. & Ettlinger, G. (1978) The effect of ablations on primary and secondary epileptic discharges in commissure-sectioned rhesus monkeys. *Electroenceph. Clin. Neurophysiol.*, 44, 23—36.

Manzoni, T., Hunter, M., Maccabe, J. J. and Ettlinger, G. (1973) Tactile discrimination performance in the monkey: the effect of commissure section on transfer of training between the hands. *Cortex*, 9, 40–55.

Mihailović, L. T. & Ćupić, D. (1971) Epileptiform activity evoked by intracerebral injection of anti-brain antibodies. *Brain Research*, 32, 97–124.

Moffett, A. M., Driver, M. V., St John Loe, P. & Ettlinger, G. (1970) Tactile discrimination performance in the monkey: the effect of unilateral posterior parietal discharging lesions. *Cortex*, 6, 68–86.

Nie, V., Upton, A. & Ettlinger, G. (1973) Behavioural impairment in the monkey following implantation of aluminium hydroxide on the temporal cortex: the role of cortical destruction. *Exper. Neurol*, 40, 632–51.

Nie, V. & Ettlinger, G. (1974) Ablation of the primary of infero-temporal epileptogenic focus in rhesus monkeys with independent secondary spike discharges. *Brain Research*, 69, 149–52.

Nie, V., Maccabe, J. J., Ettlinger, G. & Driver, M. V. (1974) The development of secondary epileptic discharges in the rhesus monkey after commissure section. *Electroenceph. Clin. Neurophysiol.*, 37, 473–81.

Ridley, R. M. & Ettlinger, G. (1973) Visual discrimination performance in the monkey: the activity of single cells in infero-temporal cortex. *Brain Research*, 55, 179–82.

Ridley, R. M. Hester, N. S & Ettlinger, G. (1977) Stimulus- and response-dependent units from the occipital and temporal lobes of the unanaesthetised monkey performing learnt visual tasks. *Exp. Brain Research*, in press.

Scheibel, M. E., Crandall, P. H. & Scheibel, A. B. (1974) The hippocampal-dentate complex in temporal lobe epilepsy: a Golgi study. *Epilepsia*, 15, 55–80.

Scheibel, M. E. & Scheibel, A. B. (1968) On the nature of dendritic spines—report of a workshop. *Communications in Behavrl. Biol. A*, 1, 231–65.

Stamm, J. S. & Pribram K. H. (1960) Effects of epileptogenic lesions in frontal cortex on learning and retention in monkeys. *J. Neurophysiol*, 23, 552–63.

Stamm, J. S. & Pribram, K. H. (1961) Effects of epileptogenic lesions of inferotemporal cortex on learning and retention in monkeys. *J. Comp. Physiol Psychol*, 54, 614–18.

Stamm J. S. & Warren, J. M. (1961) Learning and retention by monkeys with epileptic implants in posterior parietal cortex. *Epilepsia*, 2, 229–42.

Ward, A. A. (1969) Chronic foci in animals and man. In *Basic Mechanisms of the Epilepsies* (ed. H. H. Jasper *et al*) Boston: Little, Brown 263–88.

Westrum, L. E., White, L. E. & Ward, A. A. (1965) Morphology of the experimental epileptic focus. *J. Neurosurg*, 21, 1033–46.

INSANITY AND EPILEPSY IN THE NINETEENTH CENTURY

G. E. Berrios

Introduction

Eliot Slater's paper describing the association between epilepsy and psychosis has become a classic. Its historical section, however, touches mainly upon the German contribution; no mention is made of the earlier French writing which inspired the former.

This short historical paper, written expressly to pay tribute to Slater's outstanding contribution to psychiatry, is intended to fill this gap by showing how most of the logical possibilities combining epilepsy and insanity had been worked out by the turn of the century. This paper is about the history of the link between epilepsy and the psychoses mainly in nineteenth-century French psychiatry. It will illustrate how competing theories on the aetiology of epilepsy controlled views on the nature of the link and how this led to wider conceptual developments. For in trying to make sense of the link, nineteenth-century psychiatrists postulated notions such as 'masked epilepsy', 'combined psychoses' and 'hybrid or composed psychoses', which gave rise to a general question unanswerable at the time: can two different psychoses coexist in the same individual?

The beginnings

The *Dictionnaire des sciences médicales,* summarizing medical knowledge at the beginning of the nineteenth-century, was published in 1815 in Paris. The entry on 'Epilepsie' by Esquirol stated, 'Epilepsy, compounded by insanity, never gets better'.* This opinion, the last of twelve he listed, was to control European thinking on the association between epilepsy and insanity for decades. Esquirol found that four-fifths of his female inpatients with epilepsy were affected by

*All translations are the author's

monomania, mania, dementia, fury, idiocy and character disorders. The first three tally well with our present-day concept of
psychosis.

Esquirol's conclusions did not remain unheeded and in 1825, in
one of the earliest issues of the *Archives Générales de Médecine,*
Bouchet and Cazauvieilh (1825) published the results of their
enquiry into the nature of the link. The inquiry contains the first
published association between temporal lobe pathology and
insanity; five of the cases with both conditions had involvement of
the 'cornes d'Ammon'. The authors did not point this out, however, and the concept of psychomotor epilepsy had to await another
50 years before Hughlings Jackson rendered it into a clinical entity
(Jackson, 1888). Bouchet and Cazauvieilh claimed that past research.
'had been based on the assumption that epilepsy was the cause of
insanity. We shall try to analyse all the possibilities of the relationship'.

They were referring to transient ictal or peri-ictal psychotic states:
'Many patients do not become psychotic until a number of years
have passed: In some cases the psychosis appears after the fourth or
fifth admission separated by intervals in which they are well'.

Detailed post-mortem descriptions are included of epileptic,
epileptic with insanity, and insane patients. Similar lesions in the
three groups were found and the conclusion drawn that there was a
'similarity in the pathology of both conditions'. After Bouchet and
Cazauvieilh the view was held in France that no fundamental
difference existed between epilepsy and psychosis.

Theirs should be considered the first scientific account of the
nature of the link, namely, that the clinical association is not due to
a cause–effect relationship, epilepsy causing insanity, but that both
conditions have their own but related pathology. They were postula-
ting a coexistence based on the fact that the same pathological
process could produce epilepsy or insanity according to whether it
invaded the white or the grey matter. This is the way in which the
editor of the 1835 *Dictionnaire* understood Bouchet and Cazauvieilh's
contribution: 'The authors have tried to demonstrate the relationship between epilepsy and insanity . . . They suggest that both are . . .
due to phlegmasia [inflammation] of the brain, the one of the white,
the other of the grey matter' (Garimond, 1878).

This conclusion reflects two important assumptions of early
nineteenth-century neurophysiology, that the highest motor station
was subcortical and that grey matter or cortex was the seat of
consciousness or the mind (Young, 1970). Convulsions could be
explained by a pathological process impairing subcortical struc-
tures whereas insanity could be explained by processes damaging
the cortex.

These assumptions, however, tallied better with neurophysiological speculation than with clinical facts. They could not explain why grand mal seizures, although accompanied by loss of consciousness, reflecting cortical involvement, were not always complicated by insanity. Furthermore post-mortem studies had shown that cortical pathology was often absent in grand mal epilepsy.

The chance association hypothesis

This anomaly led to the acceptance of a second theory of epilepsy known as the 'reflex theory' (Temkin, 1971) after Marshall Hall who successfully introduced the concept of 'reflex' into nineteenth-century British neurophysiology (Fearing, 1930; Canguilhem, 1977). The theory stated that loss of consciousness was a secondary phenomenon produced by diminished blood supply to the cortex a physiological rather than a structural phenomenon (Temkin, 1971).

Theodore Herpin in *Du pronostic et du traitement curatif de l'épilepsie,* (Herpin, 1852) reported a series of 300 private patients none of whom had ever been admitted to a mental hospital. He observed that although long-term insanity had complicated a few cases, psychiatric symptoms were transient and only ictal or peri-ictal. A similar view was advanced by Reynolds in 1861: 'There is not, therefore, any special mental condition necessarily involved in the idea of epilepsy' (Reynolds, 1861).

Esquirol and Bouchet had carried out their statistical work on psychiatric hospital populations where a high association between insanity and epilepsy was to be expected. Herpin and Reynolds on the basis of their experience with out-patients postulated that it was due to a chance association. Insanity and epilepsy were bound to coincide in a few cases which, sooner or later, would be collected in asylums. Garimond commented when referring to this period: 'It is understandable that psychiatrists, because they make their observations in asylums, tend to generalize about the association between epilepsy and insanity' (Garimond, 1878).

The refinement of clinical descriptions

Falret reviewed the problem in 1860. He denied claims that all epileptic cases must have psychiatric complications although he accepted that: 'Epilepsy is a condition of the brain which often brings in its wake mental disorder' (Falret, 1860). His concern was threefold: sharpening clinical description of the mental state of epileptics; detecting associations between those and the epileptic phenomena themselves; and, developing criteria for forensic work.

The first problem that Falret tried to solve was clinical definition. Before Kraepelin's synthesis a large number of clinical syndromes had qualified as insanity. The fleeting presence in various combinations of hallucinations, delusions, bizarre behaviour, and obsessions was sufficient to generate different diagnostic categories. No search for a specific deep structure underlying the multifarious surface combinations was attempted. Nor indeed was the natural history of the disease considered relevant for diagnostic purposes: symptom clusters were not followed to see whether they remained true to form. Accounts of insanity often boiled down to descriptions of kaleidoscopic, transient, unstructured syndromes, with no guarantee that the next episode would resemble the previous. This was particularly so in the insanities described as associated with epilepsy. Before Falret writers only occasionally bothered to separate ictal phenomena, many of which were acute confusional states or direct seizural manifestations, from the more lasting, stable and recognizable insanities which appeared in the absence of epilepsy.

Two reasons can be given to explain why. The notion of acute confusion or delirium, as a manifestation of cerebral insufficiency, had not been recognized. The acute organic psycho-syndrome was considered by the nineteenth-century psychiatrists as yet another form of insanity (Chaslain, 1895). The concept of insanity as 'psychosis', a disease entity which ran true to form and was recognizable in successive episodes, had not been fully developed.

Falret classifies epileptic psychiatric syndromes into three groups: (1) peri- and intra-ictal mental epiphenomena; (2) interictal character changes; and (3) long-term insanities. He described the latter thus: 'Finally there are those phenomena of longer duration constituting true madness, whose onset should be described as either associated with or independent of any seizural manifestations'. In the third and last section Falret deals with the legal implications of his clinical position and supports Zachias's rule that insanity pleas should be valid only within three days of a genuine seizure, either before or after. Falret's contribution is important because he threw his weight behind the school of thought which claimed a real link between epilepsy and psychosis.

Morel and the 'Masked Epilepsy' concept

Morel, in a series of papers in the 'Gazette Hebdomadaire', put forward a radically new concept, that of 'épilepsie larvée' or 'masked epilepsy' (Morel, 1860). This concept is akin to the 'anxiety equivalent' or 'depressive equivalent' fashionable in our own century. Morel argued that epilepsy could manifest itself as convulsions, absences etc., or in abnormal mental states or abnormal behaviour. A diagnosis of 'masked epilepsy' could therefore be made in the absence of any history of convulsions. It is sufficient, he claimed, to recognize clinical features such as a paroxysmal nature and pre-morbid personality.

To advance his notion of 'masked epilepsy', Morel used the concept of epileptic character. Morel was a mental hospital psychiatrist experienced with chronic epileptics who had severe personality disorders. The adjectives used to describe the 'epileptic character' form a long list: sticky, obequious, explosive, unpredictable, over-religious, irritable, vindictive, and so on. Lecce and Caraffa (1964) have shown that most of these terms were coined during this period and provided Morel with a descriptive set. But the same descriptive set could identify insane patients who had never suffered from epilepsy. It was this group which Morel assumed to have 'masked epilepsy'.

The concept was never fully accepted in French psychiatry and after twelve years of theoretical uneasiness an important debate broke out at the Société Médico-Psychologique in 1872 (Société Médico-Psychologique, 1873). The debate was about the clinical significance of the concept and its applicability. Those who criticized it (like Fournet) insisted on the fundamental difference between the two conditions and the fallacy of diagnosing as epileptic a patient who had never had a seizure. When challenged Morel, who died in 1873 before the debate was over, produced his diagnostic 'signes'; (1) marked instability of character; (2) increased motor activity; (3) polymorphic delusions; (4) sudden, explosive behaviour; (5) episodic repetition of stereotyped insanity; (6) sudden shouting.

From then on the notion of 'masked epilepsy' declined rapidly in French psychiatry. Its obituary was written one hundred years ago by Garimond who showed both the conceptual difficulties it had given rise to, its negligible explanatory power and limited clinical value (Garimond, 1878).

The British view
The impact of the French debate in Britain will be mentioned mainly in relation to Hughlings Jackson who by 1875 had already made a reputation with his views on epilepsy. In a paper in the famous but short-lived *West Riding Lunatic Asylum Medical Reports* he wrote:

> I believe that according to some, I believe most, alienist physicians, that degree of it which is called epileptic mania, although it usually occurs after a fit, does not always do so. It sometimes 'replaces' a fit. A patient who is subject to ordinary epileptic attacks may on this hypothesis have as it were instead a paroxysm of mania. There is what is called the masked epilepsy, described by Falret [sic] . . . I used to adopt the hypothesis of masked epilepsy. But I do not now think it possible that a nervous discharge at all comparable in degree to that

which causes convulsion would cause ... epileptic mania ... I now think that another hypothesis is preferable. I think it probable that there is a transitory epileptic paroxysm in every case. (Jackson, 1875).

Jackson's view was accepted by most but did not go unchallenged. Clouston crisply wrote: 'I do not agree with Hughlings Jackson that, in cases of petit mal and slight convulsions, the explosion, not finding vent in a motor form, is more apt to extend up into mental centres' (Clouston, 1887). But he was well aware of the close association between the two conditions as his comments show:

> When I speak of epilepsy causing insanity and mental symptoms, you must clearly understand that the whole series of symptoms, bodily and mental, may in some cases be the combined result of a general disturbance of function or disease of the brain, neither the convulsions being the primary disease, nor the mania, but both being equally effects of the same cause. It is usual for the epileptic insanity not to follow at once the first appearance of fits. Most commonly years elapse before it comes on (Clouston, 1887).

But this explanation of the association is suspiciously close to Bouchet's 60 years earlier:

> It will be observed that all those relationships point to a close connection between the locus in quo of epilepsy and the seat of mental disturbance. The fact that they are related to each other in such various ways is the strongest proof of the *nearness of their pathological seat*. (Clouston, 1887).

Likewise Maudsley, in the 1879 edition of *The Pathology of Mind,* accepts the notion of 'masked epilepsy' and separates off the chronic paranoid forms: 'In the less acute and more partial forms of epileptic insanity there are commonly chronic hallucinations; the person hears distinctly a voice which insults him or commands him peremptorily to do some deed' (Maudsley, 1879).

The problem was still unresolved in British psychiatry by the turn of the century. In Tuke's *Dictionary* there are two entries on this topic. One, by James Anderson from the National Hospital entitled 'Epilepsies and insanities' is a rambling and long-winded attempt to develop Jackson's views (Tuke, 1892). The other, entitled 'Epilepsy and insanity' by Geo. Savage summarizes well the knowledge available at the time. He includes a description that strongly reminds one of Landolt's views: 'Patients, having been relieved or cured of the fits, have from that time begun to degenerate mentally and we have elsewhere described cases in which epileptiform, if not epileptic, fits have been followed by mental improvement' (Tuke, 1892).

The Question of the 'Combined Psychoses'

As a reaction to the almost total identification of epilepsy and insanity that Morel had attempted in the 1880s the French once again opted for the 'random combination hypothesis'. Thus Magnan, in his 1880 paper on 'the coexistence of various forms of insanity in the same individual' tackled the problem of the link in an entirely different way: 'Some patients suffer from both epilepsy and partial madness, mania or melancholia. These two conditions remain independent although they can influence and modulate each other' (Magnan, 1880).

This claim is as important in the solution it puts forward as in the questions it raises. For Magnan generalized and then asked 'Can two psychoses coexist in the same individual?' If so, would they influence each other in their symptomatic manifestations? If not, why can they not? What is so specific or unique about psychoses that two cannot be found in the same person at the same time?

Posing this question requires at least two assumptions. One that psychoses are stable over time, the other that there is a known cause. Magnan did assume both. Before Kraepelin, Magnan defined in his own category of 'délire chronique' the notion of psychosis as a condition which ran true to form (Magnan, 1887). Likewise he never hesitated to use heredity as an explanation. As Meeus said years later: 'The coexistence of two psychoses in the same patient was considered by Magnan to be due to double inheritance. One of the parents transmitting epilepsy and the other insanity' (Meeus, 1908).

The German contribution

The German contribution developed in the context of the German debate concerning the 'combined psychoses' or, as the title of Gaupp's classical paper expressed it, 'Zur Frage der kombinierten Psychosen' (Gaupp, 1903). This debate dealt with the question of (1) whether psychoses could become grafted upon mental subnormality or acquired brain lesion; (2) whether two psychoses could coexist in the same individual; and (3) whether the coexistence happened simultaneously or successively. The question of combined psychoses is germane to this paper and its discussion here does not constitute a departure from the central theme. It is relevant because *historically* it was discussed in association with the epileptic insanity issue and because the latter was often used as an example of two 'combined psychoses'.

The Germans started from the premise that the combination of psychoses was a real one as it occurred at a rate higher than chance (Samt, 1875). But what mainly exercised German psychiatrists at the time was the nature of the link. Buchholz wrote that epilepsy paved the way for insanity by weakening the resistance of the brain (Buchholz, 1895). Ziehen opted for a psychological account of the link claiming that the delusional system in epileptic insanity was the result of the combination of the fragmentary and fleeting insane experiences occurring during the ictal episodes (Ziehen, 1902), the theory that has been mistakenly attributed to Pond (Betts *et al.*, 1976).

It was Krafft-Ebing who first addressed himself to the problem of the 'combined psychoses'. In his book he dealt both with the question of psychoses grafted upon pre-existing mental retardation and with the coexistence of two psychoses, each preserving its individuality (Krafft Ebing, 1888). Along the same lines Ziehen had described the 'zusammengesetzte Psychosen' to which he dedicated a chapter of his *Psychiatrie* in 1902 (Ziehen, 1902). These 'composite psychoses' were constituted by grouping 'simple psychoses' such as mania, melancholia, stupor and paranoia. 'Composite psychoses' were 'periodic' like the manic-depressive psychosis, or 'non-periodic' such as Kahlbaum's catatonia, with all 'simple' components coexisting within the same episode.

Wernicke also accepted the existence of these 'composite psychoses' and said they were more common than the 'simple forms'. He renamed 'gemischten Psychosen' those 'hybrid' forms in which the two coexisting psychoses were not true to form as a result of pathoplastic interaction (Wernicke, 1900).

It is against this background, where a need for simplicity can already be detected, that Kraepelin brought about his supreme effort of synthesis by reducing the multifarious field of simple and composite psychoses to what can be called 'the two supercomposite insanities', dementia praecox and manic-depressive insanity. This he did by developing a structural view of these two forms of insanity that transcended clinical features and relied heavily on integrating factors such as natural history, prognosis and aetiology.

Equally relevant is the contribution of Erwin Stransky, the Viennese psychiatrist, who in 1906 published his 'Zur Lehre der kombinierten Psychosen' (Stransky, 1906). In this paper he rejected the view that the term 'combined psychoses' should be freely applied to any symptom-cluster. He defined the former:

> As a combination of two completely unrelated psychoses occuring simultaneously or in sequence with symptoms that have no known connection with each other, e.g. the combination of manic-depressive insanity and paranoid illness or the former with dementia praecox.

In a review in 1908, Meeus, from the Gheel Colony, reinforced this view: 'I cannot see any theoretical contradiction in the fact that, in the same individual or brain psychoses clinically different can succeed each other at short or long intervals' (Meeus, 1908).

Conclusions

Thus, by the early 1900s possible combinations linking epilepsy and psychosis had been explored in theory:

(1) The link as a chance combination
    (a) as the result of defective statistics (Herpin, 1952)
    (b) as the result of chance genetic combination (Magnan, 1880)

(2) The link as real
    (a) epilepsy producing psychoses
        (i) by weakening the brain (Buchholz, 1895)
        (ii) by disrupting reality testing (Ziehen, 1902; Gaupp, 1903)
    (b) psychosis producing epilepsy (Clouston, 1887)
    (c) both being the result of a common organic factor (Jackson, 1875)

These combinations exhaust the theoretical possibilities. That this is the case does not reduce the enormous importance of Slater's contribution. It is one thing to extrapolate from a few clinical observations and work out theoretical combinations as the masters of the past did; quite another to subject hypotheses to statistical testing. But we must not exaggerate the conceptual or clinical differences between us and the nineteenth-century either. There are good reasons to believe that textual analysis of classical writing may well yield clinical riches.

Between 1900 and 1978 the debate as to which of the possibilities mentioned above corresponds to the clinical facts continued and yet another possibility has been added; that the treatments used to cure epilepsy may be responsible for the psychotic complication. The pendulum has oscillated twice since. Glaus (1931) reported a lower incidence of epilepsy, 1.3 per thousand, among 6,000 schizophrenics than the expected incidence of epilepsy in the general population. This observation led him to conclude that epilepsy and schizophrenia were antagonistic. It has been claimed that this provided Sakel and Meduna with their rationale to use induced seizures in the treatment of the psychoses. Lennox has since quoted Sakel as rejecting this account of the rationale of his insulin coma.

The second swing of the pendulum took place when Bartlet (1957), Pond (1957) and Dongier (1959) confirmed an increased probability of psychotic states in epilepsy. In 1963 Slater and his co-workers published their work showing that a form of schizophrenia-like psychosis was associated with temporal lobe epilepsy which was different from the run-of-the-mill schizophrenia because it had no higher genetic load than the control population. It was characterized by warm and appropriate affect and was not followed by typical deterioration (Slater *et al.*, 1963).

Although the existence of the link has not gone unchallenged, (*vide* Stevens, 1966) the 1970s have seen increased efforts to corroborate the findings. Flor Henry (1976) and Betts (1974) have produced evidence showing an association between epilepsy, specifically temporal lobe epilepsy and the psychoses and a laterality effect. A schizophrenia-like psychosis is associated with dominant hemisphere pathology, affective psychosis is linked to the non-dominant hemisphere.

References

Bartlet, J. E. A. (1957) Chronic psychosis following epilepsy. *Am. J. Psychiat.*, **114**, 338–43.

Betts, T. A. (1974) A follow up study of a cohort of patients with epilepsy admitted to psychiatric care in an English city. In *Epilepsy* (ed. P. Harris and C. Maudsley). Edinburgh: Churchill-Livingstone.

Betts, T. A., *et al.* (ed.) (1976). Psychiatry. In Laidlaw and Richeus, *A Textbook of Epilepsy*. Edinburgh: Churchill-Livingstone, p. 178.

Bouchet & Cazauvieilh (1825–1826) De l'épilepsie considérée dans ses rapports avec l'aliénation mentale. Recherche sur la nature et le siège de ces deux maladies. *Arch. Gen. Med.,* **9**, 510–42; **10**, 5–50.

Buchholz (1895) Über die chronische Paranoia bei epileptischen Individuen. *Habilitationsschrift.*

Canguilhem, G. (1977) *La formation du concept de réflexe aux XVII et XVIII ème siècles.* Paris: Vrin, p. 132.

Chaslain, Ph. (1895) *La confusion mentale primitive: stupidité, démence aigüe stupeur primitive.* Asselin et Houzeau.

Clouston, T. S. (1887) *Clinical Lectures on Mental Diseases.* London: J. & A. Churchill.

Dongier, S. (1959) Statistical study of clinical and electroencephalographic manifestations of 536 psychotic episodes occuring in 561 epileptics between clinical seizures. *Epilepsia.*, **1**, 117.

Esquirol (1815) Epilepsie. In *Dictionnaire des Sciences Médicales.*

Falret, J. (1860–1861) De l'état mental des épileptiques. *Arch. Gen. de Méd.,* V Série, **16**, 661–79; **17**, 461–91; **18**, 423–43.

Fearing, F. (1930) Reflex action. In *A study in the history of physiological psychology.* Baltimore: Williams and Wilkins, p. 128.

Flor Henry, P. (1976) Epilepsy and psychopathology. In *Recent Advances in Clinical Psychiatry 2* (ed. K. Granville-Grossman). Edinburgh; Churchill-Livingstone.

Garimond (1878) Contribution à l'histoire de l'épilepsie. *Annales Médico-Psychol.* 5^{e}s, **19**, 5,181.

Gaupp (1903) Zur Frage der kombinierten Psychosen. *Centralblatt f. Nerv. und Psych.,* p. 766.

Georget (1835) Epilepsie. *Dictionnaire de Médecine ou Répertoire Général des Sciences Médicales* (2nd edn), Vol. 12. Paris: Bechet, p. 172.

Glaus, A. (1931) Ueber Kombinationen von Schizophrenie und Epilepsie. *Zeitschrift für die Gesamte Neurologie und Psychiatrie,* **135**, 450–500.

Herpin, Th. (1852) *Du pronostic et du traitement curatif de l'épilepsie.* Paris.

Jackson, J. H. (1875) On temporary mental disorders after epileptic paroxysms. *West Riding Lunatic Asylum Medical Reports,* **5**, 240.

Jackson, J. H. (1888) On a particular variety of epilepsy. *Brain,* **11**, 179.

Krafft Ebing (1888) *Psychiatrie,* Vol. 3, Stuttgart.

Lecce, C. & Caraffa, T. (1964) Evoluzione del concetto di epilettoidismo *Riv. Neurobiol,* **10**, 123–145.

Magnan, J. J. V. (1880–1881) De la coexistence de plusieurs délires de nature differente chez le même aliéné. *Arch. Neurol.,* **1**, 49.

Magnan, J. J. V. (1887) Considérations générales sur la folie. *Le progrès médical 2nd S,* 5, 190.

Maudsley, H. (1879) *The Pathology of Mind.* London: Macmillan.

Meeus, F. (1908) Epilepsie et délire chronique. Contributions à l'étude des psychoses combinées. *Ann. med. psychol., 9ᵉS,* 7, 353–382.

Morel, B. A. (1860) D'une forme de délire, suite d'une surexcitation nerveuse se rattachant a une variété non encore décrite d'épilepsie (épilepsie larvée). *Gazette Hebdomadaire de médecine et de chirurgie,* 7, 773–5; 819–21; 836–41.

Pond, D. A. (1957) Psychiatric aspects of epilepsy. *J. Indian. med. prof.,* 3, 1441.

Reynolds, J. R. (1861) *Epilepsy.* London: Churchill, p. 43.

Samt, P. (1875) Epileptische Irreseinsformen. *Arch. für Psychiatrie,* 5, 393–444; 6, 110–216.

Slater, E. *et al.* (1963) The schizophrenia-like psychosis of epilepsy *Brit. J. Psychiat.* 109: 95.

Société médico-psychologique (1873) De d'épilepsie larvée. *Annales médico-psychol.,* 5 Series, 9, 139; 155; 281; 301; 490; 493.

Stevens, J. R. (1966) Psychiatric implications of psychomotor epilepsy. *Arch. gen. Psychiat.,* 14, 461–71.

Stransky, E. (1906) Zur Lehre der kombinierten Psychosen. *Allgem. Zeitschrift für Psycho.,* 63, 73.

Temkin, O. (1971) *The Falling Sickness* (2nd edn). Baltimore: Johns Hopkins Press.

Tuke, D. H. (1892) *Dictionary of Psychological Medicine* (2 vols). London: J. & A. Churchill.

Wernicke, K. (1900) *Grundriss der Psychiatrie.* Leipzig, p. 459.

Young, R. M. (1970) *Mind, Brain and Adaptation in the 19th century.* Oxford: Clarendon Press, p. 111.

Ziehen, Th. (1902) *Psychiatrie.* Leipzig, p. 542.

METHODOLOGY

STATISTICAL AND LOGICAL THEORIES OF PROBABILITY PERTINENT TO GRIDS

P. Slater

It may seem perfectly reasonable to stipulate that a grid should be reliable and significant if important decisions depend on the results from it—for instance if the diagnosis or treatment of a patient is concerned. Moreover, the array of data in a grid, giving an informant's evaluations of a set of elements in terms of a set of constructs, is the same in its general form and in most of its mathematical properties as a two-way table giving the scores of a group of subjects on a battery of tests—the subjects correspond to the elements and the tests to the constructs. So why should not the reliability and significance of both kinds of array be investigated by the same methods?

They cannot. The reason is that the theory from which psychometric methods for measuring reliability and significance are derived assumes that samples can be drawn at random from an objectively defined population. The assumption can be satisfied by the nomothetic data in a table of test scores but not by the idiographic data in a grid.

A typical occasion for giving a battery of tests to a group of subjects occurs when their scores are needed for allocating them to different educational courses or different duties in a large organization. Before the tests can be put to such use, their reliability and significance should be investigated thoroughly. An applicant's scores should characterize him as a person, not just record a temporary state of mind. The norms for the courses or the duties should be known, and the differences between them shown to be highly significant. Then it would be possible to estimate from the candidate's scores what is his probability of adapting successfully to each of the alternative situations and hence to decide which is the best one for him (or whether he is unfitted for any).

To find out whether a test in the battery is reliable it should be given twice, with a reasonable time in between, to a random sample of the population from which applicants come. The correlation between the scores on the two occasions, which is the measure of the test's reliability, will be an unbiased estimate of the correlation in the population, provided the sample is a random one. For the same reason the norms for the courses or duties should be obtained from random samples of the people who have adapted successfully to them, if not from the records of everyone who has done so; the proof that the norms vary significantly would be invalid if they were obtained from unrepresentative samples. All these investigations need to be completed before the battery of tests is ready for use in the selection procedure.

No such preliminary investigations can be carried out when a grid is constructed specially for one informant on one occasion. The setting is likely to be a clinic, the interviewer a consultant and the informant a patient who presents some psychological problem. The clinician and the patient will collaborate in constructing the grid, with the problem as its focus of interest. Eliciting the elements and the constructs and filling in the grid will be one continuous process. The results will be wanted as soon as possible. The clinician will probably discuss them with the patient and agree on their interpretation.

Since an idiographic grid refers to a population of elements which cannot be defined objectively or sampled at random, the data for assessing its reliability and significance could not be obtained even if there was time to spare. But besides, there is not the same need for an assessment. The grid does not serve the same purposes as a battery of tests. Its primary interest is in what it shows directly, the informant's state of mind at the time of interview. Its predictive value for estimating what is to be expected in another case or on another occasion may not need to be considered, and constructs which register changes in mental states may be more suitable for inclusion in it than ones that record stable personality traits. Thus the criteria of significance and reliability proposed by statistical theory are inappropriate for it as well as inapplicable.

Must the evidence be discarded because it does not conform to statistical canons? We seem to be faced by the dilemma: if the orthodox statistical theory of probability is sound the scientific status of grid technique is questionable; if the technique is acceptable, the theory is called into question. In that case, however, there is no need to question the theory as a whole, but only its application to idiographic grids.

It has long been recognized that statistical methods are limited in their application and that probabilities have often to be estimated on the basis of evidence of other kinds. Suppose, for instance, someone is charged in court with committing a crime. Statistical evidence that people like him commit similar crimes in similar circumstances will not be admitted in evidence, no matter how high the probability they establish. Only evidence unambiguously proving or disproving the defendant's personal connection with the crime will satisfy the court. While the case is in progress and the evidence is being presented, the probability that he will prove innocent fluctuates perceptibly.

Keynes achieved remarkable success in his original attempt (1921) to develop a logical theory of probability which could be extended to such contingencies. But the problem of defining the most reasonable estimate is formidable when the evidence cannot be evaluated by reckoning up instances. Though protracted studies of the subject have been made since (notably by Carnap, 1971) no methods have yet been found for quantifying logical probability with the neat mathematical expressions, $P < .05$ etc., which have become the hallmarks of acceptable psychological papers.

Even supposing that arguments of a statistical kind can be adduced for expecting that grids are generally reliable, provided they satisfy certain conditions, whether mathematical or psychological, the proposition that a particular idiographic grid is reliable, in a particular case, must remain open to doubt. And it cannot be decided by statistical evidence; what is needed is evidence that is logically relevant. It must establish definite connections between the contents of the grid and what is known about the informant from other sources or can be verified by further investigations. We should recognize that, if such evidence is logically valid, it pre-empts the call for statistical tests.

References

Carnap, R., *et al.* *(1971) Studies in Inductive Logic and Probability.* University of California Press.

Keynes, J. M. (1921) *A Treatise on Probability.* London: Macmillan.

TWO-PHASE SAMPLING
AND COMMUNITY SURVEYS

W. Edwards Deming

Purpose

A study will be conducted to estimate the overall proportion of people that are affected with some defined psychopathology. The final determination of the psychiatric and other medical characteristics of a person will be made by a psychiatrist. A plan to use the services of trained interviewers to screen and separate into two classes (with and without apparent psychopathology) a large preliminary sample in order to conserve the time of the psychiatrist, by letting him test mainly cases that are almost surely afflicted with psychopathology, is appealing wherever the cost per case is much lower for the screening than for the psychiatric examination. It is not generally appreciated, however, that the screening-test, to be economical, must be relatively cheap and must admit only a low proportion of false negatives. This principle is not new, but illustrative calculations that show how false negatives affect costs, and why false positives are not so important, are hard to find in the literature (Kish, 1965).

Guidance in any problem comes from calculations based on the appropriate theory. The purpose here is to present some theory and a simple illustration encountered in recent practice. The conclusions drawn here will be valid within a moderately wide band of conditions that border on those used here for illustration. Conditions far afield from those studied here might require fresh calculations by use of the appropriate costs and proportions in the equations that follow, or in modifications thereof.

The conclusions drawn here are worthy of consideration in the inspection of industrial product, in situations where the final test is relatively very expensive, and where a cheap screening test can be contrived.

It is presumed that a demographic screening has already taken place in which a roster is made of each family by age of person.

People of age 60 or over can be serialized. These serial numbers constitute the frame.

The statistical procedure for screening (sometimes called two-phase sampling) may be described briefly in two steps.

Step 1 (first phase). Screening. Draw from the frame a preliminary sample of N $prime$ people. Interview by a cheap test every person in the preliminary sample. Allot each person interviewed to one of two strata:

Stratum 1: negative on screening (no psychopathology indicated).

Stratum 2: positive on screening (psychopathology indicated).

Step 2 (second phase). Psychiatric interviews. A psychiatrist interviews samples from both strata. His decisions are final. Some people in Stratum 1, the psychiatrist will find, are pathologic. These are false negatives. Conversely, he will find that some people put into Stratum 2 are in his judgement not pathologic. These are false positives.

The final sample for the psychiatrist is drawn partly from Stratum 1 and partly from Stratum 2. The selections from each stratum are made by simple random sampling, one person at a time. Textbooks on statistical procedures describe two main ways to draw for the psychiatrist a sample of people from the two strata: (1) proportionate allocation; (2) Neyman allocation.

We calculate also, for comparison, the amount of information to be expected from a plan that uses no screening at all. There is no preliminary sample in this plan: the psychiatrist interviews the entire sample.

We shall see that the distinction between proportionate allocation and Neyman allocation is important only if the screening is highly reliable, and that the best procedure may be no screening at all.

As we shall see, the proportion $p1$ of false negatives in Stratum 1 is critical. The proportion $q2$ of false positives in Stratum 2, on the other hand, is not critical, though it must not get out of hand.

In the ideal situation, there would be no psychopathology in Stratum 1 and nothing but psychopathology in Stratum 2. Interviews by the pssychiatrist would yield identical results. This goal can of course not be achieved: there will in practice be false negatives in Stratum 1 and false positives in Stratum 2.

It would be easy to construct a system of screening that would hardly ever put positive psychopathology into Stratum 1. It is only necessary to specify that a person that exhibits in the screening a shred of evidence of psychopathology shall be placed in Stratum 2. Such a procedure could easily get out of hand: the proportion $q2$ of false positives in Stratum 2 would reach an alarming proportion and would raise costs, defeating the purpose of screening. We now proceed with the calculations, in order to learn what is the best practice.

Notation

P_1 the expected proportion of cases placed in Stratum 1 in Step 1
P_2 the expected proportion of cases placed in Stratum 2 in Step 1
p_1 the expected proportion of false negatives in Stratum 1
q_2 the expected proportion of false positives in Stratum 2
p the proportion of pathologic in the entire frame
$\hat{p}$ an estimate of p

We define q_1 and p_2 so that $p_1+q_1=1$ $p_2+q_2=1$
n_1 the number of persons selected from Stratum 1 for the final sample (for examination by the psychiatrist)
n_2 likewise for Stratum 2
$n_1+n_2=n$ the size of the final sample (for the psychiatrist); n will depend on the plan adopted
$\sigma_1{}^2=p_1q_1$ the expected variance between people in Stratum 1
$\sigma_2{}^2=p_2q_2$ the expected variance between people in Stratum 2
$\sigma_w{}^2=P_1\sigma_1{}^2+P_2\sigma_2{}^2$ the average variance between sampling units within strata
$\bar{\sigma}_w=P_1\sigma_1+P_2\sigma_2$ the average standard deviation between sampling units within strata
$\sigma{}^2=P_1P_2(p-p_1)^2$ the variance between the means of the two strata
N' the number of people screened (the preliminary sample)
c^1 the cost to screen one person
c_2 the cost for the psychiatrist to interview one person.

The relative proportions of the two strata in any one study give the estimates $\hat{P}_1$ and $\hat{P}_2$ of P_1 and P_2. Step 2 gives the estimates $\hat{p}_1$ and $\hat{q}_2$ of p_1 and q_2. Then

$$\hat{p} = \hat{P}_1\hat{p}_1+\hat{P}_2\hat{p}_2 \tag{1}$$

will be an unbiased estimate of the overall proportion p that are pathologic in the entire frame.

$\hat{P}_1$ and $\hat{P}_2$ come from the preliminary sample, the screening: they are the proportions in the two strata. $\hat{p}_1$ and $\hat{p}_1$ come from the psychiatric interviews.

A 2×2 diagram may be helpful. The psychiatric interviews separate Stratum 1 into two groups with proportions p_1 and q_1, and separate Stratum into two groups whose expected proportions will be p_2 and q_2.

Psychiatric interview	Screening	
	Stratum 1	Stratum 2
No psychopathology	P_1q_1	P_2q_2
Psychopathology	P_1p_1	P_2p_2
Total	P_1	P_2

We now examine the variance of $\hat{p}$ under the three possible methods for selection of the final sample from the preliminary sample.

Proportionate allocation

In this procedure, we draw, for the final sample, the same proportion of people from Stratum 1 as from Stratum 2.

$$\left.\begin{array}{l} n_1 = n\hat{P}_1 \\ n_2 = n\hat{P}_2 \end{array}\right\} \tag{2}$$

When the results are in, we form by eqn (1) the estimate $\hat{p}$ of p. For this plan

$$\text{var } \hat{p} = \frac{\sigma_b^2}{N'} + \frac{\sigma_w^2}{n} \tag{3}$$

The optimum relation between n and N' for proportionate allocation is

$$\text{opt } n/N' = \frac{\sigma_w}{\sigma_b} \sqrt{\frac{c_1}{c_2}} \tag{4}$$

Neyman allocation

Here, we aim at the allocation

$$\left.\begin{array}{l} n_1 = n\sigma_1 P_1/\bar{\sigma}_w \\ n_2 = n\sigma_2 P_2/\bar{\sigma}_w \end{array}\right\} \tag{5}$$

Once the study is completed, we again use eqn (1) to form $\hat{p}$, for which

$$\text{var } \hat{p} = \frac{\sigma_b^2}{N'} + \frac{(\bar{\sigma}_w)^2}{n} \tag{6}$$

The optimum relation between n and N' in Neyman allocation is

$$\text{opt } n/N' = \frac{\bar{\sigma}_w}{\sigma_b} \sqrt{\frac{c_1}{c_2}} \tag{7}$$

Any non-zero sizes of, sample n_1 and n_2 for the psychiatrist, when used in eqn (1), will give an unbiased estimate of p. One of our aims here, however, is to find the optimum relationship between n_1, n_2 and N'. This we do by use of eqns (2), (4), (5) and (7). Use of samples other than the optimum indicated in the tables would yield less information per unit cost than the optimum sizes will yield.

We introduce now specific numbers for our calculations. We use $q_2 = 0.1$, and choose a few values of p and p_1. For costs, we set $c_1 = \$5$ and $c_2 = \$45$; then $c_1 : c_2 = 1/9$ and by eqns (3) and (6).

$$\text{Proportionate sampling opt } \frac{n}{N'} = \frac{\sigma_w \cdot}{\sigma_b} \sqrt{\tfrac{1}{9}} = \tfrac{1}{3} \frac{\sigma_w}{\sigma_b} \tag{8}$$

$$\text{Neyman allocation} \qquad \text{opt } \frac{n}{N'} = \tfrac{1}{3} \frac{\bar{\sigma}_w}{\sigma_b} \tag{9}$$

The total cost of Steps 1 and 2 will be

$$K = 5N' + 45n = n(5N'/n + 45) \tag{10}$$

wherein n and N' are specific to the plan adopted.

The amount of information in an estimate $\hat{p}$ was defined by Sir Ronald Fisher as

$$I = 1/\text{var } \hat{p} \tag{11}$$

The efficiency of the procedure that delivers the estimate $\hat{p}$ was defined by Morris Hansen as

$$I/K = \frac{1}{K \text{ var } \hat{p}} \tag{12}$$

which is the amount of information per unit cost for no screening at all,

$$\operatorname{var} \hat{p} = \frac{\sigma^2}{n} = \frac{p(1-p)}{n} \tag{13}$$

$$K = \$45n$$

$$I/K = \frac{1}{45p\,(1-p)} \tag{14}$$

All the above formulas are in any book in statistical theory.

We should emphasize that it is the ratio $c_1{:}c_2$ and not the absolute costs c_1 and c_2 that are important for the relationship between n and N'. Moreover, as the ratio $c_1{:}c_2$ appears only under the square-root sign, the relationship between n and N' is not very sensitive to the costs within a moderate range of $c_1{:}c_2$.

Costs in absolute numbers as necessary in order to compare the efficiency of proportionate allocation or Neyman allocation with a plan that uses no screening at all. Costs in absolute numbers are also necessary for prediction of the total cost of a study, once the plan is decided.

The calculations are shown in Tables 1 and 2. The important lines in the tables are lines 15, 21 and 24, which compare the amount of information per unit cost for the three plans under consideration. The tables also show the optimum relationships between the sizes of the samples N', n_1, n_2 under proportionate allocation and Neyman allocation.

Conclusion from the calculations
Comparisons of I/K, the amount of information per unit cost for the three plans—screening with proportionate allocation for the final sample; screening with Neyman allocation for the final sample; no screening at all—leads to the following conclusions, which are valid over moderate intervals above and below the proportions and costs that the calculations were based on.

(1) The proportion p_1 of false negatives in Stratum 1 is critical in consideration of choice of plan.
(2) Screening is most effective in the reduction of costs when the overall proportion p of the disease under investigation is low, and when the screening is highly successful in the separation of cases, leaving the proportion p_1 of psychiatric cases very low in Stratum 1, while holding the proportion of q_2 of non-psychiatric cases to a moderately low level in Stratum 2.
(3) There is little choice between proportionate allocation and Neyman allocation in drawing the final sample from the preliminary sample, unless the screening finds 85 per cent or more of the psychiatric cases and places them in Stratum 1. Neyman allocation creeps ahead of proportionate allocation as the screening improves beyond this point.
(4) Lines 11, 12, 17 and 18 in the tables show that for best efficiency (optimum balance) most of the cases for the final interviews will come from Stratum 1 unless the screening is extremely effective. This seems

Table 1. *Results of calculation, where $p = 0.1$, $\sigma^2 = 0.09$, $q_2 = 0.1$, $\sigma_2^2 = p_2 q_2 = 0.09$ and $\sigma_2 = 0.3$*

Item	p_1					
	0.15	0.10	0.05	0.025	0.01	0.005
1 $P_1 = (P_2-p)/(p_2-p_1)$	Not applicable		0.9412	0.9143	0.8989	0.8938
2 $P_2 = 1-P_1$			0.0588	0.0587	0.1011	0.1062
3 $\sigma_1^2 = p_1 q_1$			0.0475	0.0244	0.0099	0.0050
4 σ_1			0.2179	0.1561	0.0995	0.0701
5 $\sigma_w^2 = P_1\sigma_1^2 + P_2\sigma_2^2$			0.0500	0.0300	0.0180	0.0140
6 σ_w			0.2236	0.1732	0.1342	0.1183
7 $\bar\sigma_w = P_1\sigma_1 + P_2\sigma_2$			0.2228	0.1685	0.1198	0.0949
8 σ_b^2			0.0400	0.0600	0.0720	0.0760
9 σ_b			0.2000	0.2449	0.2683	0.2757
Proportionate allocation						
10 $N' = n\,(\sigma_w/\sigma_b)\sqrt{c_1:c_2}$			2.683n	4.242n	6.000n	6.990n
11 $n_1 = nP_1$			0.941n	0.914n	0.899n	0.894n
12 $n_2 = nP_2$			0.059n	0.086n	0.101n	0.106n
13 var $\hat p$			0.0649/n	0.0441/n	0.0300/n	0.0249/n
14 K, total cost	58.42n	66.21n	75.00n	79.95n		
15 $I/K = 1/K$ var $\hat p$	0.264	0.342	0.444	0.503		
Neyman allocation						
16 $N' = n\,(\bar\sigma_w/\sigma_b)\sqrt{c_1:c_2}$			2.693n	4.362n	6.721n	8.716n
17 $n_1 = n\sigma_1 P_1/\bar\sigma_w$			0.921n	0.847n	0.747n	0.660n
18 $n_2 = n\sigma_2 P_2/\bar\sigma_w$			0.079n	0.153n	0.253n	0.336n
19 var $\hat p$			0.0645/n	0.0421/n	0.0251/n	0.0177/n
20 K, total cost	58.46n	66.81n	78.61n	88.58n		
21 $I/K = 1/K$ var $\hat p$	0.265	0.355	0.508	0.637		
No screening						
22 var $\hat p = \sigma^2/n = p(1-p)/n = 0.09/n$						
23 K $= 45n$						
24 $I/K = 1/K$ var $\hat p$ $= 0.247$						

reasonable on reflection, because Stratum 1, intended to be pure, no psychopathology, will otherwise contain far more psychopathology than Stratum 2.

Remarks
The calculations shown here indicate that screening (or two-phase sampling) may not pay off unless the cost c_1 is considerably smaller than c_2. A rough break-even point for the ratio $c_1:c_2$ is about 1:6. The ratio $c_1:c_2$ is likely to be especially low when the screening and classification are to be done on the basis of records, and where the final investigation may require costly fieldwork or costly interviews. In some of my own experience with perusal of records on hand for screening and stratification, with interviews by a psychiatrist in the

Table 2. *Results of calculation, where* $p = 0.2$, $\sigma^2 = 0.16$, $q_2 = 0.1$, $\sigma_2{}^2 = p_2q_2 = 0.09$ *and* $\sigma_2 = .3$

Item	p_1					
	0.15	0.10	0.05	0.025	0.01	0.005
1 $P_1 = (P_2-p)/(p_2-p_1)$	0.9333	0.8750	0.8235	0.8000	0.7865	0.7821
2 $P_2 = 1-P_1$	0.0667	0.1250	0.1765	0.2000	0.2135	0.2179
3 $\sigma_1{}^2 = p_1q_1$	0.1275	0.0900	0.0475	0.0244	0.0099	0.0050
4 σ_1	0.3571	0.3000	0.2179	0.1561	0.0995	0.0705
5 $\sigma_w{}^2 = P_1\sigma_1{}^2+P_2\sigma_2{}^2$	0.1250	0.0900	0.0550	0.0375	0.0270	0.0235
6 σ_w	0.3536	0.3000	0.2345	0.1936	0.1643	0.1533
7 $\bar\sigma_w = P_1\sigma_1+P_2\sigma_2$	0.3533	0.3000	0.2324	0.1849	0.1423	0.1205
8 $\sigma_b{}^2$	0.0350	0.0700	0.1050	0.1225	0.1330	0.1365
9 σ_b	0.1871	0.2646	0.3241	0.3500	0.3647	0.3695
Proportionate allocation						
10 $N' = n (\sigma_w/\sigma_b) \sqrt{c_1:c_2}$	1.587n	2.646n	4.146n	5.422n	6.659n	7.231n
11 $n_1 = nP_1$	0.933n	0.875n	0.823n	0.800n	0.786n	0.782n
12 $n_2 = nP_2$	0.067n	0.125n	0.177n	0.200n	0.214n	0.218n
13 var $\hat p$	0.147/n	0.116/n	0.080/n	0.060/n	0.047/n	0.042/n
14 K, total cost	52.94n	58.23n	65.73n	72.11n	78.30n	81.15n
15 $I/K = 1/K$ var $\hat p$	0.128	0.147	0.189	0.231	0.272	0.291
Neyman allocation						
16 $N' = n (\bar\sigma_w/\sigma_b) \sqrt{c_1:c_2}$	1.589n	2.649n	4.184n	5.679n	7.689n	9.199n
17 $n_1 = n\sigma_1 P_1/\bar\sigma_w$	0.943n	0.875n	0.722n	0.675n	0.550n	0.458n
18 $n_2 = n\sigma_2 P_2/\bar\sigma_w$	0.057n	0.125n	0.228n	0.324n	0.450n	0.542n
19 var $\hat p$	0.147/n	0116/n	0.079/n	0.056/n	0.038/n	0.029/n
20 K, total cost	52.94n	58.23n	65.92n	73.39n	83.44n	91.00n
21 $I/K = 1/K$ var $\hat p$	0.129	0.147	0.192	0.244	0.319	0.374
No screening						
22 var $\hat p = \sigma^2/n = p(1-p)/n = 0.16/n$						
23 K	= 45n					
24 $I/K = 1/K$ var $\hat p$	= 0.139					

field, the ratio $c_1 : c_2$ has run in the neighbourhood of 1:40, or even 1:100.

The tables indicate that there is no economy to realize from screening unless it be sufficiently effective to render $p_1 \leqq \frac{1}{4}p$. The proportion q_2 of false positives in Stratum 2 deserves reasonable care, but under conditions in any way similar to those studied here, is nowhere near as critical as the proportion p_1 of false negatives in Stratum 1.

A sample designed for Neyman allocation by use of a value of p_1 that turns out to be wide of the mark may end up with greater variance than proportionate allocation. Proportionate allocation is foolproof and simple to apply (Deming, 1960; Hasel, 1954).

Unfortunately, the more reliable be the screening, the more difficult it is to measure how good it is.

One might summarize the conclusions from the equations and the tables by saying that, in the absence of sound information about the screening and a clear indication that proportionate or Neyman allocation would pay off, it is perhaps best to use no screening at all. If screening be adopted, it is best to use proportionate allocation unless there be a firm basis for Neyman allocation.

In addition to the guidance supplied by the equations, there are some arguments to bear in mind about screening that are not expressible mathematically. Some of these arguments are negative on screening; some are positive. I may remind the reader first on the negative side that use of screening (unless the screening be carried out on the basis of records collected in a previous study) requires a second interview (the one by the psychiatrist) of the people that are selected into the final sample. There is always the possibility that this second appointment may encounter resistance and loss of the psychiatric interview. This means a total loss of the case, except for information of secondary importance that was already elicited in the screening interview. The loss from refusals at the second interview undoubtedly varies widely between communities, and with public interest in respect to the disease under investigation. Resistance may be serious in one place and not in another.

A further negative point to bear in mind is that screening necessitates some extra administrative attention in the fieldwork. Besides, with screening, there is the selection of the final sample to accomplish. These costs are in the equations, supposedly incorporated in the symbol c_1, but the equations do not take care of the circumstance in which the organization is small and over-worked, with no-one to take on with diligence the extra duties involved.

On the positive side of the ledger, also not in the equations, is the insight that a preliminary sample yields about the material in the frame, and about the problems that one will encounter in the investigation. A fairly large preliminary sample, even though the equations do not indicate any economical advantage of screening, puts before the investigator a miniature display of the frame. One will often find in this display problems that on-one could otherwise foresee. It may bring out, for example, cases that do not belong in the investigation at all. It may bring out the existence of difficult cases. It may indicate errors in the delineation of sampling units, and need of more care in preparation. In a preliminary sample of hospital records intended for an investigation of adults 21 to 60, the preliminary sample contained admissions of age 20 and under. There were also cases beyond the intended age-limit, and emergency cases of various kinds not intended for investigation. Some cases were transfers from other hospitals, and would require requests for additional notes. Without the preliminary sample, the investigators would have had no warning that 15 per cent of the frame was made up of a spectrum of blanks to be discarded, nor that 10 per cent of the frame came from transfers. A fairly large preliminary sample, screened by use of the case-notes, permits one to throw out the blanks and to stratify the valid cases by type of ailment indicated. The final sample for further study may then be balanced in the main categories of hospital diagnosis (Gurland, Deming and Kuriansky, 1974).

Sampling to measure the prevalence of a rare characteristic is a subject all by itself, beyond the scope of this paper, and must be dismissed here with the statement that for a characteristic that has a high probability of being treated in an institution, samples might be taken from clinics and hospitals, accompanied by a sample from the general population. Statistical procedures to determine with a prescribed probability that the prevalence of a certain rare disease does not exceed some small proportion such as $p \leq 1/50$ call forth still further theory, also not to be covered here.

This paper should also mention circumstances that often face investigators in small research organizations where there is a shortage of psychiatrists or of men with other specialized knowledge. It is then imperative to carry out screening. In fact, the optimum plan in such circumstances may be to use a preliminary sample that is double or treble the size that the equations indicate; then to adjust the sizes n_1 and n_2 of the final sample by proportionate allocation or by Neyman allocation, holding $n_1 + n_2$ to the maximum number that the psychiatrists can handle. The information per unit cost will be less than that indicated by the optimum ratio of N' to n, but it will be valid statistical information bought at the lowest price consistent with the restraints.

Note in respect to the tables
The symbol n in Tables 1 and 2 has a different meaning from one panel to another. Thus, the number n required to reach a given precision with proportionate allocation would not be the same number required to reach the same precision with Neyman allocation, oir with no screening at all. Comparison between plans is possible only in lines 15, 21 and 24 which show the efficiency I/K of the plans, wherein n does not appear.

Acknowledgements
I am indebted to my friend and colleague Dr Morris H. Hansen for many important suggestions on this paper, and for the good fortune

to work with him on several studies that have required the use and extension of the theory presented here. It has also been my good fortune to work with Dr Barry Gurland of the new York State Psychiatric Institute, under whose direction a number of studies have required consideration of screening and allocation of sample.

References

Deming, W. Edwards (1960). *Sampling Design in Business Research*. New York: Wiley. p. 295

Deming, W. Edwards (1972). Some theory on the influence of the inspector and environmental conditions. *Statistica Neerlandica,* **26,** 3, 101–12.

Hase, A. A. (1954). Problems in inventory. In O. Kempthorne (editor), *Statistics and Mathematics in Biology* (ed. O. Kempthorne). Iowa State College Press, p. 267

Kish, L. (1965). *Sampling Techniques*. New York: Wiley, p. 407

Gurland, B. Deming, W. Edwards and Kuriansky, J. (1974). On trends in the diagnosis of schizophrenia. *American Journal of Psychiatry,* **4,** 402–8.

Tepping, B. J. & Bailar, B. A. (1968) Effects of interviewers and crew leaders. *Series ER No. 7. Washington: Bureau of the Census.*

PERSONAL IMPRESSIONS

ELIOT SLATER AS SEEN BY A CONTEMPORARY

Desmond Curran

I have probably known Eliot Slater longer than any other contributor to this *Festschrift*. We did not know each other at Cambridge. We first met just over 50 years ago. This was at St George's Hospital in 1925. I had gone there in 1924, so he came a year later. But we only really got to know each other well when we met again at the Maudsley in 1931. We have kept in touch ever since. I greatly treasure his friendship.

I was struck in re-reading the fascinating 'autobiographical sketch' and moving 'retrospect' that he has contributed to the impressive volume of his selected papers*, by certain similarities in our early training and experiences, completely different though the outcome has been; for Eliot is surely the most original and productive British psychiatrist of his generation, with an international reputation based not only on the famous more general textbooks he has written with others, but also upon his other contributions with special reference to genetic research; and, of course, I can make no such claim.

I must first apologize in advance if, in what follows, I bring myself in too much; I am under orders to indulge in reminiscences; so I do not see how that can be avoided. It will also become clear that I have found myself at variance with Eliot on certain points. But I know him well enough to be sure that he will not mind in the least. I have also little doubt that any future argument will end by my finding 'I have no loophole left to stand a leg on' (a metaphor in which I proudly claim a proprietary interest, since it once sprang unbidden from my lips; so far as I know it is original).

St George's Hospital
I know I am prejudiced, since I spent so much of my working life

---

*Man, Mind, and Heredity. Selected Papers of Eliot Slater on Psychiatry and Genetics. Edited by James Shields and Irving I. Gottesman. Johns Hopkins Press. Baltimore and London: 1971.

associated with the hospital. But when I took Eliot to task because in his 'autobiographical sketch' I thought he was describing the students in our day as well-dressed youths who were excellently taught in the sort of medicine and manners required in their subsequent careers as successful, if at times sycophantic, fashionable West End general practitioners (a well-known breed in those—for some—more prosperous times, when the world of 'Upstairs Downstairs' still persisted) he replied: 'I am sorry if what I wrote sounded hard. If I am convicted of exaggerating the facts, I did not exaggerate the impression made on me at the time ... Actually, I dearly loved St George's, and was most reluctant to leave. I was always delighted that I went to what was then a small medical school, with medical students who behaved like gents and not ruffians ('beefy and boisterous') and a tradition for tolerating individualities, even eccentrics'.

I remember Eliot well as a student. He stood out as quite different. He has forgotten. Whereas all the other students *did* wear short white jackets, Eliot wore a much longer confection of a café au lait colour. I recall him with his then red hair (which he wore rather long, in those days uncommon), falling over his forehead, absorbed in reading Proust, quite oblivious of his surroundings, his absorption punctuated by an occasional quite loud yelp of laughter. He was tall, pale and lanky, perhaps rather aloof, but it was obvious to all of us fellow students that he had a first rate brain and was very well read. He was perhaps thought a bit unusual, but none the worse for that. We all liked him very much.

I know that I am now going to invite the editorial blue pencil, but I am pretty sure that St George's between the wars was unique in Great Britain as a medical school in its combination of small size, pleasant atmosphere, and excellent clinical teaching for undergraduates. What follows may also possess some interest as illustrating the changes that have occurred in the medical and psychiatric scene, with special reference to a budding psychiatrist.

There had been no preclinical department at St George's since 1905, when it was closed for what seems now strange reasons. The annual intake was only 20–25, many from 'Oxbridge' and the rest from King's in the Strand. With few exceptions, the students, housemen and consultants were not only civilized and friendly, but intelligent and conscientious. We would all mix together with delightful informality in the primitive students' club luncheon room, with marble-topped tables, apparently the first in any London teaching hospital. It certainly looked it. Little store was set by set lectures. And, indeed, when I first came for interview, I was accepted by the then Dean with the words 'Personally, I think nearly all lectures are a bloody waste of time. But do come and see for yourself'. All the 'firms' were small, seldom more than 3–4. This was admirable for instruction in the personal examination of patients (I am speaking of physical examination). Much emphasis was laid on small group tutorials. The housemen got bed and board but no pay, and the visiting consultants were of course 'honorary'. There were no professors. The only full-time members of the staff that I can remember were the pathologist (a dim, dull, droning Scot, later a professor elsewhere), and a biochemist (a fat man whose speciality was lipid metabolism). On the wall of the pathology laboratory hung a real sacred cow in a glass case, with the inscription 'The skin of the Cow from which the first vaccine matter was taken by Dr. Jenner. Presented by his family'. Jenner had been one of the first students of the New Medical School attached to St George's in the eighteenth century where he was a pupil of John Hunter 1770–1772.

I am sure that patients in our day received kindly attention and excellent nursing in the often rather beautifully proportioned wards with good window spacing, but with deplorable sanitary annexes. I recall with pleasure the pleasing custom of giving champagne—or any other drink they preferred—to the dying. We had by a long way the largest alcoholic cost per patient of any London hospital, the table of figures being published bitterly by some temperance society, and republished with glee in the *Hospital Gazette* in 1936.

The administrative staff consisted of the Hospital Secretary, dressed in a morning coat, and assisted by, I think, two clerks, who tapped away at, I think, the only two typewriters in the place. How different from nowadays, when admistrators are, like committees and subcommittees, 'spawned with the fertility of a herring'.

Our system of teaching, essentially by apprenticeship, did work very, very well at that time. I was told by a later Dean, who went into it, that we had the best examination results of any London medical school. And to confute Eliot, far from becoming fashionable West End general practitioners, quite recently (1963) a photograph was found and published in the *Hospital Gazette* of the 16 members in my time in the 'Cottage', the name for the residents' quarters. All but one, and he was a part-time anaesthetist, subsequently became consultants, and two of them, Leslie Hilliard (later a leader in the field of mental subnormality) and myself subsequently became psychiatrists. Others of our near contemporaries, like Eliot, and the attractive fey bohemian, Bill Hubert (the joint author of the well known East–Hubert Report on the psychological treatment of crime), did the same; and several others I remember as well.

So that later when we met at the Maudsley, in 1931, three of the nine Assistant Medical Officers came from St George's.

The only instruction in psychiatry that we had were a few lecture demonstrations of a *Grand Guignol* type in a mental hospital by our

'Lecturer on Insanity'. He was not a member of the hospital consultant staff. The hospital did not have any consultant psychiatrist. I do not know what deductions, if any, can be drawn.

Eliot clearly enjoyed his time at St George's and from his own account blossomed in that urbane and friendly atmosphere after feeling rather the odd man out at Cambridge. This was in spite of the fact he had the misfortune to be House Surgeon to the one real boor on the staff. Nor was the consultant to whom he was House Physician of much help; he was apparently stupidly discouraging.

I, on the other hand, had the great good fortune to be House Physician to Anthony Feiling, charming and cultured, always immaculate, and with the courtesy, manners and appearance of what, even then, seemed a bygone age. He was a good general physician, but primarily a neurologist. He played the major part in the initiation and later expansion of psychiatry at St George's. Personally, I am deeply grateful to him for many things. He died in 1975 aged 89.

Before we met again at the Maudsley in 1931, both Eliot and I had postgraduate experience as residents in neurological hospitals and in unsatisfactory mental hospitals, but in the reverse order. In addition, I had the chance of working at the Phipps Clinic at Baltimore with Adolf Meyer.

My experience of neurologists is different from Eliot's. I have not come across much anti-psychiatric feeling, or have not been aware of it. At the Maida Vale Hospital for Nervous Diseases, Edward Mapother, whom later I was to succeed there, was, amongst his many other activities, the visiting psychiatric consultant. There were also a number of psychotherapists, one of them the most gifted I have known, if the criterion for that is doing good to his patients, rather than in contributions to psychopathological theory. Mapother offered me a job at the Maudsley on my return from the Phipps, having first, with Tony Feiling, wangled a travelling fellowship to go there.

Again, I disagree with Eliot over Adolf Meyer and his 'psycho-biology', which I think has been much maligned by him. I fully realize that to read many of Adolf Meyer's papers produces the uneasy feeling that one's mind is slipping. But he did *not* disregard the importance of making a diagnosis (to be replaced by 'dynamic understanding') or of constitutional and genetic factors. Fundamentally, I do not see much difference between what Meyer taught and the 'multidimensional diagnosis' to which 'clinical psychiatry' so warmly subscribes, except in the clarity of exposition in the latter, and the Swiss-Germanic fog that renders impenetrable so much of what Adolf Meyer has written. I think perhaps you had to fall under the spell of the magician by sitting at his feet. All my contemporaries at the Phipps—the seniors including Horsley Gantt and Curt Richter in their labs, and the outstanding 'intern' with me, Harold Wolff—greatly admired Adolf for his compassion, tolerance, great learning, breadth of outlook and deep respect for each patient's unique individuality. The 'Meyerian miasma' did not adversely affect these distinguished men in their productivity.

The Maudsley
I hope this digression on 'psychobiology' will be forgiven. Anyway, owing to this experience, I did not find the Maudsley quite such a startling revelation as Eliot did, according to his autobiographical sketch. At Maida Vale, I had known both Mapother and the don-like, disdainful Golla, the one the Medical Superintendent of the clinical side and the other Director of the Laboratories. Golla once said to me, 'Dickens? He writes about such *crude* people.' Golla had stayed on the staff at Maida Vale to keep his hand in clinically. He was, with Grey Walter, a pioneer in the introduction of the electro-encephalograph for clinical use. But sometimes his own clinical judgement faltered. I am credibly informed he once diagnosed an almost purely Welsh-speaking Welshman with multiple sclerosis as 'an interesting case of jargon aphasia'.

We, the juniors on the clinical side, as already mentioned, were then a small group of about nine, only to increase gradually. There were no registrars. So the total medical staff were greatly outnumbered by the inpatients, which I am told is no longer true. We also had to carry a heavy load of outpatients both at the Maudsley and at outlying clinics, which I am told is no longer true either. Instead of perhaps two or three new outpatients per session, we had to see up to eight or more, as well as old patients.

As Eliot has rightly pointed out in his autobiographic sketch, we were all devoted to Edward Mapother and I would also entirely agree that Aubrey Lewis was the leading spirit amongst us juniors. He was even then very learned; nor did he hide this under a bushel. I remember many years later saying to a distinguished Scandinavian psychiatrist that 'existentialism' quite baffled me. What were the tenets of the faithful? He replied: 'It is really quite easy. If you put up any proposition you will get the reply "No, that is wrong".' If this is correct, Aubrey was an early leading exponent.

I recently re-read a book, given by the author to my parents in 1893, because I remembered it contained an essay on euthanasia, one of Eliot's later interests. This book also contains recollections of conversations held in 1882 with the well-known Oxford don and Rector of Lincoln College, Mark Pattison, which, if slightly modified, and with some drops from Adolf Meyer's 1933 Maudsley Lecture added, may give a picture of the sort of discussion battles that went on so often between our two leading disputants at the Maudsley in those very happy far-off days of long ago. Looking back, we were all pretty vocal.

The subject was whether Englishmen were, on the whole, better off in the reign of George II than either before or since:

Aubrey Lewis: I shall not be committed. But I *might* predict that England will go on declining.

Eliot Slater: I insist that, in discussing the question, we must start with the assumption that there is more good than evil in life.

Aubrey: I don't see why I should assume anything of the sort. I think I shall take up the view of Schopenhauer.

Eliot: May I recall to you some of the conclusions that may be drawn from that wildly antisocial theory? For example, might not those persons who say they would not, if they could, live their lives over again—in other words that, so far as their experience goes, the good of life is a *minus* quantity—ought not these Schopenhauerites to rejoice instead of sorrowing at the sight or news of a fatal car smash?

Aubrey. Well, suppose that I do grant that life is good on the whole, what relevance has that to human progress?

Eliot: For convenience of figures, let us compare the present time with the time when the population of England was one-third of what it now is, and let us suppose that the average Englishman was twice as happy as now. Even on this extreme supposition, the aggregate of happiness in England would be half as great again now as then: Englishmen in tripling their numbers, would have gained more collectively than they have lost individually.

Aubrey: (impatiently) But that is not what is generally meant by progress. You must define your terms. But first you should read Froschhammer's tactful reservation on your naive and uncritical apparent espousal of Neo-Darwinism, and Roux's Entwicklungs-mechanik—that means roughly mechanics of evolution you know and —and—

Eliot: You suggest I am wrong. What did your authorities conclude and what do *you* mean by progress?

Aubrey: (huffily) I really cannot be expected to give a succinct answer to a problem that is inherently complex and difficult.

Eliot: And pray what problem would you not put in that category?

Aubrey: I should advise you to make a start with the aggressive vitalism you may find in Driesch——Do be careful with those keys and stop swinging them about like that. They might hit me.

When he came to Maudsley Eliot himself had changed a great deal outwardly. Instead of his former café au lait coloured jacket, he now constantly wore a somewhat shapeless and very hairy tweed suit of a most unusual 'love in the mist' colour. We all at once recognized his first rate mind with an unusual twist to it. Many of us were then rather sceptical of intelligence tests, but when all the junior staff were guinea pigs for a new one ('Black is to white as

Purple is to . . . ' sort of thing) I for one began to waver. Eliot came easily top, Aubrey second after a big interval, at which he was sore displeased, and then the rest of us all bunched together after another big interval. I was one from the bottom.

Eliot did not get really going productively until after he went to study under Rüdin in Munich in 1934, but, looking back, it was striking how not only we British juniors, but the very distinguished and mature German emigrants, who arrived in 1933 escaping from the Hitler regime, at once recognized his intellectual quality and originality. Willi Mayer-Gross, Erich Guttmann and Eddie (Eduardo) Krapf whom I saw much of both then and subsequently had no doubts from the start about the quality of Eliot's intellect.

I think patients in those days may have found Eliot rather aloof and preoccupied. I think that probably, both then and later, this arose partly from the need for self-protection, surely quite commonly shown by those who are highly imaginative and sensitive and are all-too-readily upset by the sadness and injustice of this world.

Mapother was another who had no doubts. When I last saw him, in 1939, he was a sick man, breathless and in bed, but brave as always and his mind clear and incisive. I had prepared a memo with my opposite number, Macdonald Critchley, the neurologist, on our proposed plans for the development of a neuropsychiatric service in the Navy. I thought that if fit enough, to be consulted might please him, and also I knew nobody whose opinion I would value more highly. His devoted wife said 'Do come'. After some trenchant, astringent and valuable comments he began to reminisce over the staff at the Maudsley. He was sure that Eliot was the man to make the most important contributions. He also told me how he so much admired his complete and utter integrity, adding 'so unlike some of the others I could mention', which, to my great surprise, he then proceeded to do.

Post-Maudsley

Ever since Maudsley days, I have always been delighted to see Eliot, but we have never worked together as colleagues. I think I have read much of what he has written; and I have often heard him speak, which he can do admirably.

I cannot judge of his contributions on the mathematical level, since I am innumerate. It would be wholly presumptuous of me to express any opinion on the battle between the importance of a major dominant single gene as opposed to the polygenetic theory in the origin of schizophrenia. I would be quite incapable of starting. Yet I have found some of his papers left me wondering. For example, in 'Birth order and the maternal age of homosexuals' I was as sure as may be that homosexuality is not a specific propensity which you either possess or you do not; or in Kinsey's terms there is a continuum varying between his 0 and 6. Where on this continuum did the Maudsley cases diagnosed as 320.6: pathological personality: sexual deviation: homosexuality' lie? And might this not crucially affect the value of the study?

Again in the address 'Hysteria 331', it never had occurred to me since Phipps days that anybody had regarded 'hysteria' as a discrete more or less clearly defined condition, comparable to schizophrenia. When I might describe a case as 'posturing hysteria' or as showing 'hysterical amnesia' I would have just regarded this as a convenient 'shorthand' initial description, that did convey *some* meaning but needing further study for evaluation. This address rather struck me as an elegant sledgehammer to crack a non-existent nut. But I was quite wrong. Many did, and perhaps still do, regard hysteria as a 'clinical syndrome' of purely psychogenic origin.

To take some more general subjects in which Eliot has shown a keen interest. He kindly sent me a reprint of a symposium on euthanasia, in which he took part, held in 1973 by the Royal Society of Health. I was fascinated to find that the arguments for and against were almost identical with those that appeared in the *Fortnightly Review* a hundred years before in 1873 and reprinted in the volume already mentioned, except for a striking passage from Sir Thomas More's *Utopia,* in which euthanasia was gladly accepted and recognized by all. The author of the 1873 article, entitled 'The cure for incurables' also suggests the possible value of testamentary capacity as a test. If someone was capable of making a will, why should he not also be capable of deciding how soon that will should take effect? In a sense, what could be more neatly logical? And does it really differ in essentials from the 'proforma' proposed for non-resuscitation in special care units by the euthanasiasts?

But Eliot goes on to say 'From the standpoint of Society, it is the duty of the dying man to die' and backs up this proposition with cogent reasons. Later he suggests that there is no biological reason why man should not be able to look forward to dying,'not in suffering, but in a state of bliss. The pleasure centres of the brain are there only waiting to be mobilized'.

Let us sincerely hope they will be.

Now, both for personal reasons, and as the result during recent years of seeing a considerable number of seniles, mindless and incontinent, often nobly cared for by their relations (for many such cases come under the Court of Protection to which, as Lord Chancellor's Visitor, I rendered reports), I am personally in favour of legislation on euthanasia, much on the same lines as was recently proposed, and heavily rejected in Baroness Wootton's Bill. The 'medicated survival', that I have seen all-too-often, seemed to me fantastic. But, of course, the dividing line between not prolonging life 'officiously' and actively hastening death is one difficult to draw. Yet I had an uneasy feeling that Eliot's logical and compassionate plea might provoke antagonism. And doubtless the alleged origin of the sardonic smile might do the same. Apparently, the natives in Sardinia in days gone by were wont to eat such of their countrymen as were worn out by age. By his own consent, the stringy old gentleman would himself issue the invitations to the guests at this final feast, greeting them with the original prototype of the sardonic rather than blissful smile.

I certainly do not wish to seem foolishly facetious. I am quite serious, in advocating 'euthanasia', with suitable safeguards, that would ensure it was not comparable to the Nazi gas chamber. There are so many for whom death 'would be a merciful release' from any humane or reasonable standpoint.

To take another interest, penology. It is obvious that the gladiatorial system of trial in this country in courts of law is far more unpleasant for *doctors* (and their reputation) than the inquisitorial system in other countries, for reasons that need not be recapitulated. But is the latter system, on the whole, better for 'justice' than ours? That is something I just do not know.

Many of the readers of this volume will, I am sure, have greatly enjoyed 'What happened at Elsinore'. For those who were enchanted by it, as I was, may I recommend 'Horatio's Version' on the same Hamlet theme by Alethea Hayter? It is a splendid parody of the official inquiry before which witnesses are called. There had naturally been a lot of ugly rumours going about in Denmark about what had happened at Elsinore. 'King Fortinbras was most anxious that the whole truth about this very distressing affair should be fully established', as Voltimand, who had been appointed chairman, said in opening the proceedings. It has the further recommendation of giving Eliot much pleasure. I am indeed sorry that two other essays of Eliot's, both written by him for *Festchrifts,* one for Fernandez of Lisbon, and the other for Manfred Bleuler of Zurich, have appeared in journals improbably read by many. Happily, Eliot gave me reprints written in English.

In the first he argues most plausibly that Shakespeare (of Stratford) did not write Shakespeare; and whilst not claiming who did, he suggests he must have been the sort of person revealed by a study of the Sonnets. Eliot is inclined to think that the Sonnets' author did not go further than 'eyes', or at most a 'romp' with the 'lovely boy'. Personally, I find this hard to believe. But on Eliot's side is the 'mythohistorical truth' of a prize-winning sonnet in a competition for one written by Mr W.H. to Shakespeare.

Whenas—methinks that is a pretty way
To start—my father spoke to you anent
The precious po'm I got the other day,
The perfum'd posy and the pot of scent,
My drowned eyes are constantly bedewed;
The cruel rod of wrath I have not 'scaped,
My mother has been cool, my brother rude,
Honest, you'd think I was already raped
—You really think I'm like a summer's day?
Really and truly? Thank you ever so—
Behind the Globe, if I can get away,
I'll show my weals and tell thee all my woe,
In your next po'm, an thou wouldst give me joy,
Will you make clear I'm not that sort of boy?

The other essay is on the 'Colour imagery of poets' and is based more on adding up sums. I had never realized before how 'brown' was so seldom used by poets, nor quite how exotic was the colour imagery used by Gerard Manley Hopkins in his non-religious poems.

Eliot has always shown an intense and wide-ranging curiosity that happily still continues. Some men have a capacity for intense concentration; but I cannot recall anyone else who can apply this enviable endowment with such skilful imagination and ingenuity to such a wide range of interests. These include general textbooks, internationally recognized; genetic studies in various types of mental disorder and disease; clinical investigations into neurosis, psychopathy and the psychoses associated with epilepsy; statistical methodology; twin studies; more general issues affecting society and the individual, such as eugenics, penology and euthanasia; music, chess, 'pathography', and various aspects of literature, more recently Shakespeare in particular. But the list is not complete for he has written an all-too-short book of poems and made his name as an abstract painter. His selected papers, edited by others, is followed by a bibliography that, up to 1970, included 148 references to his work.

Further, although it is certainly possible to disagree, it is always quite clear what he means. If the essence of a good style, in addition to this, is 'honesty, clear thought, good manners, clear-sightedness' and 'the power to think with the heart as well as the head' Eliot has it.

I think his influence on psychiatry in Great Britain has been almost wholly beneficial. It may be difficult for a younger

---

*The late Dr C. P. Blacker (MC, GM, DM, FRCP), was a great character. He left the Maudsley not long before I came. I think he must hold a record in group therapy. He ran one for his male patients, using the technique of boxing gloves rather than verbalization. He laid one of them out for he had been a boxing blue at Oxford, and had to carry him to bed unconscious.

generation to realize, to use the late Pip Blacker's* somewhat florid language, how the inter-war years 'covered a period when yeasty growths of theory and steamy screens of narcotizing jargon were obfuscating the minds of many young men and women who beheld themselves as pioneers of new systems, creeds and revelations'. Both by his own serious works and, indirectly, as an editor he has done much to correct such dangers. Also, as the editors of the selected papers have pointed out, Eliot has rightly stressed 'the value of numerical analysis in reaching a rational judgement. All-embracing explanations and concepts are of dubious value for Slater, as for Karl Popper, since they do not permit testing and refutation'. I have read that 'as some saw it' Eliot, Willi Mayer-Gross and Martin Roth were guilty in the 1954 edition of *Clinical Psychiatry* of a 'savage and ill-informed attack on psychoanalysis'. These three would, I think, be amongst the last of the psychiatrists I have known to whom the terms 'savage and ill-informed' would be applicable. And one can only note that in the 1960 edition their former critique of psycho-analysis was curtailed, because no reply to correct and enlighten the heathen had been forthcoming.

Eliot certainly delights in controversy, but nobody I know is more genuinely pleased to be shown that he is wrong, or indeed is more naively surprised that this attitude should not be shared by others. It certainly is not. Without hesitation, I can correct Eliot on that point.

Eliot has every reason to look back with pride on his achievements. And all his old friends are proud to have known him.

NEUROPSYCHIATRIC INTERLUDE

Kenneth Davison

It is my privilege to have been Senior Registrar to Eliot Slater at the National Hospital for Nervous Diseases, Queen Square, London, from 1961 to 1964. It was intellectually a most invigorating and seminal period in my career and I am still working on some of the ideas that first germinated whilst sitting at the feet of Eliot Slater. His unit at the National consisted of only one ward of nine beds but through this passed a stream of unusual and fascinating patients. Naturally neuropsychiatric cases predominated but there was a fair selection of patients with functional psychoses and neuroses, particularly the grosser forms of hysteria. There was also an extensive out-patient commitment in which Eliot was supported by Dick Pratt, Douglas Bennett, Richard Hunter and, until his death, Joe Shorvon. Although at this time Eliot was Director of the MRC Psychiatric Genetics Research Unit he was punctilious about fulfilling his clinical commitments at the National.

The highlight of the week was undoubtedly the Thursday morning case conference. Never can patients have been assessed in such detail by so eminent a company. In addition to the clinicians mentioned above, Psychology was represented by Elizabeth Warrington and Professor O. L. Zangwill, Neurophysiology by Martin Halliday, Psychiatric Social Work by Vera Seal and Eric Glithero, Occupational Therapy by Mrs Hunter and Nursing by Sister Cookson. There were always several visitors, usually including eminent overseas guests, who contributed to the discussion. Case histories were presented by the Senior and Junior House Physicians, who were medically well-qualified trainee neurologists. The hapless House Physician would be subjected to an intensive, though good-humoured, cross-examination from Eliot that would have done credit to a Queen's Counsel. The many House Physicians' capacity to cope with this intellectual assault naturally varied and it was apparent that Eliot was not disposed to tolerate fools gladly. Nevertheless everyone had his say and Eliot was always prepared to accept reasoned arguments. Even the victims seemed to enjoy the proceedings.

At the beginning of 1963 two significant events occurred. One was the appointment of Eliot as Editor-in-Chief of the *Journal of Mental Science,* now the *British Journal of Psychiatry* with consequences of enhanced prestige for that publication and for British psychiatry that are now recognized. The second was the publication of Eliot's study, in collaboration with A. W. Beard and Eric Glithero, of the schizophrenia-like psychoses of epilepsy (Slater *et al.,* 1963). This work made a profound impression on me and triggered off an explosion of ideas which is reverberating round my head to this day. At last some sense could be made of the succession of patients with epilepsy and 'schizophrenia' who passed through the psychiatric ward at the National Hospital. In my view a significant observation was the evidence of cerebral damage in a majority and of gross cerebral lesions such as neoplasms in a proportion of the cases. In conjunction with their lack of correlation with the frequency of fits, this suggested that the psychoses were aetiologically related to the underlying cerebral lesion. An extension of this line of argument led me to suggest to Eliot that epileptic psychoses may be a special case of a general category of schizophrenia-like psychoses associated with organic cerebral disorders. Some weight was added to this argument by a striking patient with Wilson's disease and apparently typical schizophrenia then being treated in the department and previously reported by A. W. Beard (1959), one of my predecessors as Senior Registrar. Eliot's characteristic response was to suggest that I should seek data that would test the hypothesis. Accordingly I began a scrutiny of the inpatient records of the National Hospital for the decade 1954–1963 for possible examples of the combination of organic cerebral disorder other than epilepsy and 'schizophrenia' as defined by the 1957 WHO Committee (1959). Some 80 likely cases were found which, after interviewing the survivors, gathering further information and in many cases re-admitting them for detailed assessment, were eventually reduced to 44 patients who fulfilled the criteria. Excluding the 15 patients who were psychotic at the time of their first admission we were left with 29 who had developed a schizophrenia-like psychosis subsequent to their admission to the National Hospital. I calculated that, if all the patients admitted with a diagnosis indicating organic cerebral disorder other than epilepsy during the period 1954–1963 were at the age of maximum risk for schizophrenia and had survived until the end of 1963, the number of cases expected to develop coincidental schizophrenia was 13. As the observed psychoses were a minimum and the estimated psychoses were a maximum, it seemed reasonable to conclude that schizophrenia-like psychoses were developing in patients with organic brain disorders to an extent many times greater than by chance expectation. This favoured my hypothesis.

A mass of information about the physical state, phenomenology, psychometry, personality and family history of these patients, together with that of some others specially referred, was collected with the invaluable help of Vera Seal and Eric Glithero. The brain disorders concerned proved to be a remarkably heterogeneous collection, including multiple sclerosis, various congenital lesions, extra-pyramidal disorders, post-traumatic and post-infective states. A brief preliminary report has been published (Davison, 1966) but the definitive paper is still in preparation. Indeed information about these patients, particularly post-mortem reports, is still coming in. To quote the final sentence from Slater, Beard and Glithero (1963): 'It is as a mock-up of the genuine schizophrenic that the schizophrenic-like epileptic is worth special study'.

A few months after starting this work, in the course of a discussion over lunch, Eliot said he thought it would be a good idea to review the literature on this subject and asked if I would kindly do so for the *British Journal of Psychiatry*. My acceptance of this commission might not have been so casual if I had realized that it would involve examining, with the assistance of Christopher Bagley, then Research Assistant in the Department, some 1,500 references of which 782 were eventually used, and my undertaking an 'O'-level course in German. Until my proficiency in German became adequate, Eliot generously translated several monographs and articles for me. The review was eventually published as Part II of the RMPA Special Publication No. 4 (Davison and Bagley, 1969) but without Eliot's initial stimulus and persistent encouragement it would never have seen the light of day. I felt honoured when Eliot chose to use my diagrammatic representation of the hypothetical factors, including organic brain disorder, involved in the aetiology of schizophrenia, in his monumental work with Valerie Cowie on psychiatric genetics (Slater and Cowie, 1971).

Others will no doubt refer to Eliot's Olympian intellect which is so apparent in his scientific publications. I should rather emphasize his integrity and humanity which I observed at first-hand in his dealings with staff and patients. He had the capacity to inspire his staff to emulate his own high standards; how else explain the award of the Gaskell Gold Medal to four of his Senior Registrars while holding that post, surely a statistically significant series.

We have corresponded and met from time to time in the past decade, yet Eliot remains imprinted on my mind as an endearing character in a series of incidents from my period at the National Hospital: Eliot insisting on using the stairs rather than the lift to reach the sixth floor to the distress of younger but less fit colleagues;

Eliot clad in chef's hat and apron dishing up Christmas lunch to patients; Eliot being congratulated on his psychotherapeutic skill by an eminent ex-analyst; Eliot's kindness to a member of staff during her final illness. Most vivid of all is Eliot's delivery of the first Shorvon Memorial Lecture at the National Hospital in November 1964. This coincided with his resignation from the National Hospital after a disagreement with the neurological staff over the future of the Psychiatric Department. The lecture was, appropriately enough, concerned with the dangers inherent in labelling patients as hysterics, particularly by neurologists, which on its subsequent publication (Slater, 1965) provoked an uncharacteristically tetchy response from Sir Francis Walshe (1965). The most memorable feature of the occasion was, however, the remarkable demonstration in Eliot's favour by the unusually large audience. Whatever the attitude of their seniors, the junior staff of the National Hospital were determined to express their esteem and appreciation for one whose eminence they instinctively recognized and whose departure they regretted.

Fortunately, departure from the National did not signify departure from the British psychiatric scene which he continues to grace with distinction. Long may this be so.

On this felicitous occasion, this former junior colleague is grateful for the opportunity to salute his old Chief.

References

Beard, A. W. (1959) The association of hepato-lenticular degeneration with schizophrenia. *Acta Psychiatrica et Neurologica Scandinavica,* 34, 411–28.

Davison, K. (1966) Schizophrenia-like psychoses associated with organic brain disease. Preliminary observations on fifty patients. *Newcastle Medical Journal,* 29, 67–73.

Davison, K. & Bagley, C. R. (1969) Schizophrenia-like psychoses associated with organic disorders of the central nervous system: a review of the literature, Part II. (pp 113—184) In *Current Problems in Neuropsychiatry* (ed. R. N. Herrington), pp. 113–184. RMPA Special Publication No. 4, Ashford, Kent: Headley Brothers.

Slater, E. (1965) Diagnosis of 'Hysteria'. *British Medical Journal,* i, 1395–9.

Slater, E. & Cowie, V. (1971) *The Genetics of Mental Disorders.* London: Oxford University Press, p.30.

Slater, E., Beard, A. W. & Glithero, E. (1963) The schizophrenia-like psychoses of epilepsy. *British Journal of Psychiatry,* 109, 95–150.

Walshe, Sir Francis (1965) Diagnosis of hysteria. *British Medical Journal,* ii, 1451–4.

WHO Study Group on Schizophrenia (1959) Report. *American Journal of Psychiatry,* 115, 865–872.

ELIOT SLATER—A TRIBUTE

César Pérez de Francisco

I come from a family of physicians and odontologists; illness and therapeutic efforts were the background of my early life. When I was able to define and state clearly to myself what I felt, it was to realize that my father, my grandfather, my uncles, and all physicians, were combating the darker side of life. By this I mean that the war we, the white armies, wage is aimed at restoring health, at imposing order on the havoc caused by disease, and at preventing death; we are not accustomed in our work to see much of creativity, one aspect of the excellence human beings can achieve. I believe that the engineer, the farmer, the manufacturer and the miner all feel themselves to be in one way or another creative in producing, bridges, food, tooth-paste, or mercury.

But the highest aim a doctor can hope to accomplish is to recover for his patient a biological balance. Perhaps this is the basis on which the behaviour of a physician is built. He knows that man has but a poor foothold, is subject to the ravages of time and to an unavoidable transiency. He knows too, more or less clearly, the sad and tragic faces of existence. Of course, he knows also, and there is no doubt that this is an exception, the joy of birth; but even here, and using the term 'therapist' in a strict sense, he knows that to help and to deliver is not to cure. Hence, this image of the physician as antagonist of disease, pain and madness represents only one aspect of the truth about him.

When I met Eliot Slater I suspected that before me there was in Unamuno's words a complete man. Not a man all-of-a-piece, which would imply simplicity, but, a complete man in the subtle and infinite complexity that the term implies. I shall not easily forget those big high boots, for it was winter, his warm clothes of a sporting cut, harmonious, nonchalant. He saw me that first time, in the Unit to which I was to return to work after three years. It was winter in 1964 and we talked for a while. We talked of his friend of Munich days, Dionisio Nieto, now Professor of Psychiatry in Mexico, under

206

whose guidance I took my first steps in psychological medicine. All this was a long time ago but I remember that he recalled Pasternak and the translations of his poems so well done by his first wife; he talked of his children, of his second wife and, of course, of his activities and of things I could do when part of the team. The impression, at first mere conjecture, was becoming firmer: this man had a strong personality.

Compared with the many months of postgraduate clinical studies in Paris, those I spent in London in late 1967 were in marked contrast. From my first stumbling steps in psychiatry in Mexico, reading through the 'bible', Mayer-Gross, Slater and Roth, I realized that Anglo-Saxon thinking was rigorous. Upon becoming a member of the Genetics Unit, this opinion was confirmed day after day. Eliot Slater made me decide first exactly *what* it was I wanted to do. Whenever we talked, he drove me to telling him exactly *what* I meant. He made me understand exactly what research consists of. He did not present it as description, nor as criticism, nor as a difficult pursuit, but as a way of life. It consisted of attaining, first of all, small and already-known truths which when discovered by oneself, flourish again and seem virgin. To be able to read a karyotype was an accomplishment I owe to J. Khan, since he taught me how to do it, but before him, Eliot Slater, who forced me to make my own ideas clear to myself before starting any work.

His teachings were transcendant in far more than their practical aspects. I remember that for some reason I made some comments about psychopathic personalities. On realizing that there was no end to my argumentativeness, for I admit I have a marked weakness for arguments, he brought me the next day the proof-sheets of an important part of the third edition of *Clinical Psychiatry*. He would be grateful he said if I would criticize and correct the chapter. I do not have to describe how embarrassing it was for me to accept the proofs for such a purpose. But, I read them with a scientific passion, with a true eagerness to find new points to debate, so as to feed and preserve the intellectual pleasure which I gained from arguing with Eliot Slater. I never finished learning as much as I should have liked. Whether this was due to the short time I stayed at the Maudsley or to my own limitations I cannot say.

For these reasons, and because of the deep affection I feel for my English professor, I always call when visiting London. On the most recent occasion, we went to the Royal Society of Medicine's Club which used to be in Chandos House, to lunch and to talk at ease. We drank coffee in the yard warmed by a tender spring sun and then we went to the small room where he edited the *British Journal of Psychiatry*. I call this room minute when I compare it with one's mental image of such a prestigious journal. I did not accept gladly

Slater's leaving his position as Editor-in-Chief of the *Journal*. When I told him so, he gave me another lesson: 'Ten years', he said, 'is enough. Let others come and do it, let them change the whole approach, let the tone be modified, let other viewpoints evolve'—I kept my silence and listened—'Besides', he added, 'now I read a lot, I listen to music, I paint, I write poems, and some philosophical essays about science'.

I was then aware again of what I had already realized. Slater is creative in every sense of the word. He strives at all times, and here I remember Ortega's words, to *make* his life with elegance and dignity.

Many have been able to know Eliot Slater the scientist and doctor either directly, through his books, the three editions of *Clinical Psychiatry*, the volume on genetic psychiatry, and his work with William Sargant on physical treatments in psychiatry, his numerous papers or through the homage that Shields and Gottesman dedicated to him. Few know that Eliot Slater is a poet too.

In *The Ebbless Sea* (1962) he published poems written between 1922 to 1962. A wonderful book! Not only because it is proof of his creativity; but because in discovering that the psychiatrist and the scientist is also a poet we realize Slater's great intellectual restlessness. It is a good book because it shows all the flavour of a proud, intelligent being caught between the joy of living and the certainty of death. Perhaps, that is why he begins his work with the epitaph for a poet:

Stranger, smile kindly; 'twas my youth to blame
    That I once hoped that you might know my name.

It is a most difficult thing to try to understand a poet without mastering the language in which he writes. I think, however, that I have understood the implicit beauty of 'Summer', the refined and subtle humour of 'Good Resolution', and the tenderness of 'Re-encounter' where love arises from metaphysical profiles and transitoriness. Since in this book we are paying homage to a man we all love and admire, I have translated into Spanish, for him the title of his book of poems and the last poem in it.

'The Ebbless Sea' may be translated into Spanish in just one word which is, incidentally, a seaworthy one: *pleamar*. My reason for the choice are that 'ebb' means a receding sea and implies decline or loss. Since the suffix contradicts the 'ebb' we must be dealing with a desire to describe fullness. In Spanish, *pleamar* means the end or the highest part of the tide, and it means too the time such a tide lasts. It is my wish that the Spanish translation of the poems that ought some day to be made should be called *Pleamar*. Let us now pass on to those wonderful four lines which Slater has named 'Coda', which, as we know, is the name which, in music, is given to the brilliant addition to the last part of a musical piece. It has not been easy, however, to find a just and equivalent Spanish expression for 'Be not cast down'. I finally translated it as 'No te aflijas, oh Dios!'. This, then, is the result:

Coda

Be not cast down, O God! When disappear
 Thou and Thy Works, the Substance and the Law,
There was one morning of ten billion* years
 Which I, E. Slater, found without a flaw.

 No te aflijas, oh Dios! cuando desaparezcan
 Tú y Tus obras, las Sustancia y la Ley
 Hubo una mañana entre diez billones de años
 Que yo, E. Slater, hallé sin falla.

The Editors, Sir Martin Roth and my old friend Dr Valerie Cowie asked me to be brief. I mention this because I have so many more things to say. Though we have all had fine professors and skilful teachers, there are few masters. I am proud to have contributed to this book. I have been and remain Eliot Slater's pupil.

---

*10^{13}.

ELIOT—A WAR-TIME ENCOUNTER

How *Patterns of Marriage* originated in a cabmen's café at
Camberwell Green

Moya Woodside

It was in July, 1943, the fourth year of the war, that I first met Eliot. At that time, the peripatetic students of the evacuated London School of Economics Mental Health Course had returned to Cambridge for final revision and exams. Nine months previously, after our introductory lectures, we had set out from Cambridge encumbered by bicycles, typewriters, suitcases, torches, ration books and identity cards, to do our clinical psychiatry at Mill Hill Hospital, our child guidance and mental deficiency at Oxford with fire-watching included, then back to Cambridge when uncertainties about future employment began to loom large on the horizon.

One day, our senior tutor announced that 'a doctor at Maudsley' proposed to make a study of marriage and neurosis, and was looking for a psychiatric social worker to undertake the interviewing. Was anyone interested? Another student and myself said we would like to hear more about the project; and in due course, separate appointments in London were arranged.

When I arrived at the Maudsley Hospital with my introduction to 'Dr Slater', a tall, benevolent-looking gentleman appeared, spoke to me kindly, and suggested that instead of having lunch in the hospital cafeteria, we would go elsewhere. So we walked down to Camberwell Green, went into what appeared to be a sort of cabmen's shelter and there, over wartime stew and mash, followed by cups of *ersatz* coffee, Eliot expounded his ideas and aims for the study. I cannot now remember how our discussion went, but evidently my interest and enthusiasm must have outweighed my total lack of experience, since Eliot thereupon offered me the job, subject to success in the forthcoming Mental Health Certificate examination.

Little did I realize then what I was letting myself in for. Two hun-

Patterns of Marriage by E. Slater and M. Woodside, Cassell, London, 1951.

dred married soldiers from two different military hospitals in Surrey to be selected, interviewed and, more difficult, persuaded to let me interview their wives as well; a 48-item 'personality test' to be administered to both spouses. Owing to wartime industrial conscription, all childless wives were working so they had to be visited in the evening. This often involved me in journeys to remote and unknown suburbs of London in the black-out, sometimes with air-raid warnings in progress. When the flying-bomb attacks on London were at their height, interviewing of wives had to be suspended. Eliot then arranged for me to have a reader's ticket at the British Museum Library where, for a month or so, I perused the relevant literature on marriage, sex, neurosis and so on, under the disapproving surveillance of the librarian.

During the $3\frac{1}{2}$ years of fieldwork for the project, Eliot and I met regularly, often weekly, at Sutton Emergency Medical Service Hospital to go through the latest batch of interview reports and discuss any ideas or problems which came up. What I learnt and absorbed from these meetings proved an unsurpassable training for research: attitudes, methods and techniques, separation of fact from comment, avoidance of unsubstantiated statements, and always the emphasis on clear thinking and economy of expression, attributes which permeate all Eliot's work. Even when our formal partnership came to an end and I took up another appointment in America we remained in touch, shuttling chapters of our joint book (*Patterns of Marriage*) to each other across the Atlantic for comment and approval.

After my return to London some years later, Eliot was, as always, ready to encourage and advise me about any project I undertook. His guidance on the drafting and lay-out of proposed papers was particularly valuable. Surveys of such diverse groups as attempted suicides arriving at Guy's Hospital, women abortionists in Holloway Prison, and offenders on psychiatric probation in Edinburgh, all benefited from his objective criticism. Looking back over the years, I can truthfully say that the experience of working with Eliot imbued me with an irresistible commitment to research, and laid the foundation for a research career which has brought lasting professional satisfaction.

APPENDIX

*Including selected book reviews.

PUBLICATIONS OF ELIOT SLATER*

1935

1. Slater, E. The incidence of mental disorder. *Ann. Eugen.* 6: 172-86.
2. Curran, D., and Slater, E. Mental disorder in general practice: a plea for clinical psychiatry. *Lancet* 1: 69-71.

1936

3. Slater, E. German eugenics in practice, *Eugen. Rev.* 27: 285-95.
4. Slater, E. The inheritance of manic-depressive insanity. *Proc. Roy. Soc. Med.* 29: 981-90 (Section of Psychiatry pp. 39-48).
5. Slater, E. The inheritance of manic-depressive insanity and its relation to mental defect. *J. Ment. Sci.* 82: 626-34.
6. Slater, E. The inheritance of mental disorder. *Eugen. Rev.* 28: 277-84. (Reprinted in *Mental Hygiene,* 1937, 3: 28-37.)

1937

7. Slater, E. Mental disorder and the social problem group. In *A Social Problem Group?* ed. C. P. Blacker, pp. 37-49. London: Oxford University Press.

1938

8. Slater, E. Mental diseases, heredity. In *British Encyclopedia of Medical Practice,* ed. H. Rolleston, vol 8, pp. 552-63. London: Butterworth.
9. Slater, E. Zur Periodik des manisch-depressiven Irreseins [On the periodicity of manic-depressive insanity]. *Z. Ges. Neurol. Psychiat.* 162: 794-801.
10. Slater, E. Zur Erbpathologie des manisch-depressiven Irreseins. Die Eltern und Kinder von Manisch-Depressiven [On the inheritance of manic-depressive insanity: the parents and children of manic-depressives]. *Z Ges. Neurol. Psychiat.* 163: 1-47.
11. Slater, E. A critical review: Twin research in psychiatry. *J. Neurol. Psychiat.* 1: 239-58.
12. Mayer-Gross, W., and Slater, E. Psychoses. 1. Affective psychoses. In *British Encyclopedia of Medical Practice,* ed. H. Rolleston, vol. 10, pp. 267-91. London: Butterworth.

1939

13. Slater, E. Über Begriff und Anwendbarkeit der Manifestationswahrscheinlichkeit [On the concept and applicability of the probability of manifestation]. *Allg. Z. Psychiat.* 112: 148-52.

---

*Including selected book reviews.

14. Guttmann, E., Mayer-Gross, W., and Slater, E. Short-distance prognosis of schizophrenia. *J. Neurol. Psychiat.* 2 (New Series): 25-34.
15. Shrimpton, E. A. G., and Slater, E. Die Berechnung des Standardfehlers für die Weinbergsche Morbiditätstafel [The calculation of the standard error for the Weinberg morbidity table]. *Z. Ges. Neurol. Psychiat.* 166: 715-18.

1940
16. Slater, E. Professor Edward Mapother. *Character and Personality* 9: 1-5.
17. Sargant, W., and Slater, E. Acute war neuroses. *Lancet* 2: 1-2.

1941
18. Slater, E. The inheritance of twinning. *Proc. 7th Internat. Genet. Congress 1939,* ed. R. C. Punnett, p. 266 (abstract). Cambridge: Cambridge University Press.
19. Slater, E. War neuroses—General symptomatology and constitutional factors. *Med. Press and Circular* 205: 133-35.
20. Debenham, G. R., Hill, D., Sargant, W., and Slater, E. Treatment of war neurosis. *Lancet* 1: 107-109.
21. Sargant, W., and Slater, E. Amnesic syndromes in war. *Proc. Roy. Soc. Med.* 34: 757-64.

1942
22. Slater, E. Psychosis associated with vitamin B. deficiency. *Brit. Med. J.* 1: 257-58.
23. Lewis, A., and Slater, E. Neurosis in soldiers. *Lancet* 1: 496-98.

1943
24. Slater, E. The neurotic constitution. A statistical study of two thousand neurotic soldiers. *J. Neurol. Psychiat.* 6: 1-16.

1944
25. Slater, E. A demographic study of a psychopathic population. *Ann. Eugen.* 12: 121-37
26. Slater, E. Genetics in psychiatry. *J. Ment. Sci.* 90: 17-35.
27. Slater, E. The war-time development of British psychiatry. *Nevro-patologia i Psikhiatria* 13: 59-63 (in Russian).
28. Slater, E. and Slater, P. A heuristic theory of neurosis. *J. Neurol. Psychiat.* 7: 49-55.
29. Sargant, W., and Slater, E. *An Introduction to Physical Methods of Treatment in Psychiatry.* 2nd ed. 1948; 3rd ed. 1954; 4th ed. 1963, Edinburgh: Livingstone; and Baltimore; Williams and Wilkins.

1945
30. Slater, E. Psychological aspects of family life. In *Rebuilding Family Life in the Post-War World,* ed. J. Marchant, pp. 92-106. London: Odhams.
31. Slater, E. Psychological factors in cutaneous affections. *Brit. Med. Bull.* 3: 185-86.
32. Slater, E. Modern tendencies in eugenics. *Health Education J.* 3: 182-85.
33. Slater, E. Neurosis and sexuality. *J. Neurol. Nurosurg. Psychiat.* 8: 12-14.
34. Craike, W. H., and Slater, E., (with the assistance of George Burden). Folie à deux in uniovular twins reared apart. *Brain* 68: 213-21.
35. Heppenstall, M. E., Hill, D., and Slater, E. The EEG in the prognosis of war neurosis. *Brain* 68: 17-22.

36. Garai, O., (with a statistical note by Eliot Slater). Immersion as a factor in the development of hypertension. *Brit. Heart J.* 7: 200-206.

1946
37. Slater, E. An investigation into assortative mating. *Eugen. Rev.* 38: 27-28.
38. Slater, E. The modern family. *Plain View* 9: 224-30.
39. Carse, J., and Slater, E. Lymphocytosis after electrical convulsion. *J. Neurol. Neurosurg. Psychiat.* 9: 1-4.
40. Gainsborough, H., and Slater, E. A study of peptic ulcer. *Brit. Med. J.* 2: 253-58.

1947
41. Slater, E. A note on Jewish-Christian intermarriage. *Eugen. Rev.* 39: 17-21.
42. Slater, E. A biological view on anti-semitism. *Jewish Monthly* 1(8): 22-28.
43. Slater, E. Neurosis and religious affiliation. *J. Ment. Sci.* 93: 392-96.
44. Slater, E. Genetical causes of schizophrenic symptoms. *Mschr. Psychiat.* 113: 50-58.
45. Slater, E., and Slater, P. A study in the assessment of homosexual traits. *Brit. J. Med. Psychol.* 21: 61-74.
46. Mannheim, M. J., and Slater, E. The psychopathology of a correspondence column. *Brit. J. Med. Psychol.* 21: 50-60.

1948
47. Slater, E. Psychopathic personality as a genetical concept. *J. Ment. Sci.* 94: 277-82.
48. Roberts, J. A. F., and Slater, E. Genetics, medicine and practical eugenics. *Eugen. Rev.* 40: 62-69.

1949
49. Slater, E. The basic principles of psychiatry. *Nursing Times* 45: ii, 682-83.
50. Slater, E. The inheritance of twinning. *Hereditas* (Proceedings, 8th International Congress on Genetics, Stockholm, 1948), pp. 665-66 (abstract).

1950
51. Slater, E. Consciousness. In *The Physical Basis of Mind,* ed. P. Laslett, pp. 36-45. Oxford; Blackwell.
52. Slater, E. Perspectives in psychiatric genetics. In *Perspectives in Neuropsychiatry,* ed. D. Richter, pp. 173-82. London: H. K. Lewis.
53. Slater, E. Psychiatric genetics. In *Recent Progress in Psychiatry,* ed. G. W. T. H. Fleming, vol. 2, pp. 1-25. London: Churchill.
54. Slater, E. Kriegserfahrungen und Psychopathiebegriff [The experiences of wartime and the concept of psychopathy]. *Mschr. Psychiat.* 119: 207-26.
55. Slater, E. The genetical aspects of personality and neurosis. *Congrès international de Psychiatrie, Rapports VI,* pp. 119-54. Paris: Hermann.
56. Sargant, W., and Slater, E. The influence of the 1939-45 war on British psychiatry. *Congrès international de Psychiatrie, Comptes Rendus VI,* pp. 180-96. Paris: Hermann.

1951
57. Slater, E., and Woodside, M. *Patterns of Marriage.* London: Cassell.
58. Slater, E. Evaluation of electric convulsion therapy as compared with conservative methods of treatment in depressive states. *J. Ment. Sci.* 97: 567-69.
59. Hallpike, C. S., Harrison, M. S., and Slater, E. Abnormalities of the caloric test results in certain varieties of mental disorder. *Acta Otolaryng.* 39: 151-59.

1952

60. Lewis, A., and Slater, E. Psychiatry in the Emergency Medical Service. In *History of the Second World War: Medicine and Pathology,* ed. V. Z. Cope, pp. 390-407. London: Her Majesty's Stationery Office.
61. Slater, E. El estudio de los gemelos en psiquiatria [Twin study in psychiatry]. *Actas Luso-Esp. Neurol. Psiquiat.* 7: 122-34.

1953

62. Slater, E. Statistics for the chess computer and the factor of mobility. *Transactions of the Institute of Radio Engineers Professional Group on Information Theory,* pp. 150-52, 198-200. London: Ministry of Supply.
63. Slater, E. (with the assistance of Shields, J.). Psychotic and neurotic Illnesses in Twins. *Med. Res. Coun. Spec. Rep. Ser., No. 278.* London: Her Majesty's Stationery Office.
64. Slater, E. Psychiatry. In *Clinical Genetics,* ed. A. Sorsby, pp. 332-49. London: Butterworth.
65. Slater, E. Mental diseases, heredity. In *British Encyclopaedia of Medical Practice,* 2nd ed., vol. 8, pp. 543-55. London: Butterworth.
66. Slater, E. Genetic investigations in twins. *J. Ment. Sci.* 99: 44-52.
67. Slater, E. Sex-linked recessives in mental illness? *Acta Genet. (basel)* 4: 273-80.

1954

68. Mayer-Gross, W., Slater, E., and Roth, M. *Clinical Psychiatry.* London: Cassell (2nd ed. 1960; for 3rd ed., extensively rewritten, see 137.)
69. Slater, E. The McNaughten Rules and modern concepts of responsibility. *Brit. Med. J.* 2: 713-18.
70. Polonio, P., and Slater, E. A prognostic study of insulin treatment in schizophrenia. *J. Ment. Sci.* 100: 442-50.
71. Sargant, W., and Slater, E. Physical methods of treatment in psychiatry. In *Refresher Course for General Practitioners,* ed. H. Clegg, pp. 177-88. London: British Medical Association.

1955

72. Slater, E. La psychiatrie en Grande-Bretagne [Psychiatry in Great Britain]. In *Encyclopédie Médico-Chirurgicale.* Paris.
73. Slater, E., and Shields, J. Twins in psychological medicine. Paper read to the British Association, reported in *Nature (Lond.)* 176:532-33.
74. Alexander, C. H. O'd., and Slater, E. The relative strengths of the openings. *Brit. Chess Mag.* 75: 177-80.

1956

75. Elithorn, A., and Slater, E. Prefrontal leucotomy. Views of patients and their relatives. *Brit. Med. J.* 2: 739-42.
76. Shields, J., and Slater, E. An investigation into the children of cousins. *Acta Genet. (Basel)* 6: 60-79.

1957

77. Slater, E. Areas of interdoctrinal acceptance: An organicist speaks. In *Integrating the Approaches to Mental Disease,* ed. H. D. Kruse, pp. 41-43. New York: Hoeber-Harper.
78. Slater, E. The twin-study method in wider perspective: Discussion, First International Conference on Human Genetics, Copenhagen, 1957. *Acta Genet. (Basel)* 7: 20.
79. Nixon, W. L. B., and Slater, E. A second investigation into the children of cousins. *Acta Genet. (Basel)* 7: 513-32.

1958

80. Slater, E. The sibs and children of homosexuals. In *Symposium in Nuclear Sex,* eds. D. R. Smith and W. M. Davidson, pp. 79-83. London Heinemann.

81. Slater, E. The biologist and the fear of death. *Plain View* 12: 29-42. (Republished with minor revisions in 1969, as 'Death: the biological aspect' in *Euthanasia and the Right to Death,* ed. A. B. Downing, pp. 49-60. London: Peter Owen.)

82. Slater, E. The monogenic theory of schizophrenia. *Acta Genet. (Basel)* 8: 50-56.

83. Elithorn, A., Glithero, E., and Slater, E. Leucotomy for pain. *J. Neurol. Neurosurg. Psychiat.* 21: 249-61.

1959

84. Cowie, V., and Slater, E. Psychiatric genetics. In *Recent Progress in Psychiatry,* ed. G. W. T. H. Fleming, vol. III, pp. 1-53. London: Churchill.

85. Slater, E., and Meyer, A. Contributions to a pathography of the musicians: 1. Robert Schumann. *Confin. Psychiat.* 2: 65-94.

1960

86. Slater, E. Galton's heritage. *Eugen. Rev.* 52, 91-103.

87. Slater, E. Mapother memorial. VI: The psychiatrist. *Bethlem-Maudsley Hospital Gazette* 4(1): 7-10.

88. Shields, J., and Slater, E. Heredity and psychological abnormality. In *Handbook of Abnormal Psychology,* ed. H. J. Eysenck, pp. 298-343. London: Pitman Medical. (Issued by Basic Books, New York, 1961).

89. Slater, E., and Meyer, A. Contributions to a pathography of the musicians: 2. Organic and psychotic disorders. *Confin. Psychiat.* 3:129-45.

1961

90. Slater, E. Some considerations on mental health and genetic disease. In *Biological Problems Arising from the Control of Pests and Diseases,* ed. R. K. S. Wood, pp. 81-88. London: Institute of Biology.

91. Slater, E. Heredity of mental diseases. In *Clinical Aspects of Genetics* (The Proceedings of a Conference held in London at the R.C.P., 17-18 March, 1961), ed. F. Avery Jones, pp. 23-29, London: Pitman Medical.

92. Slater, E. Colère et irritabilité sont-ils des caractères essentiels de la personnalité des compositeurs allemands? [Are temper and irritability essential characteristics of the German composers?] *Vie Méd.* 42: S₃, 59-60.

93. Slater, E. The judicial process and the ascertainment of fact. *Mod. Law Rev.* 24: 721-24.

94. Slater, E. The thirty-fifth Maudsley Lecture: 'Hysteria 311'. *J. Ment. Sci.* 107: 359-81.

95. Slater, E., and Zilkha, K. A case of Turner mosaic with myopathy and schizophrenia. *Proc. Roy. Soc. Med.* 54: 674-75.

1962

96. Slater, E. Trends in psychiatric genetics in England. In *Expanding Goals of Genetics in Psychiatry,* ed. F. J. Kallmann, pp. 219-27. New York: Grune & Stratton.

97. Slater, E. Psychological aspects. In *Modern Views on 'Stroke' Illness* (Symposium held at the RSM, London, 23 January 1962), pp. 41-48. London: The Chest and Heart Association.

98. Slater, E. Birth order and maternal age of homosexuals. *Lancet* 1: 69-71.

99. Beard, A. W., and Slater, E. The schizophrenia-like psychoses of epilepsy. *Proc. Roy. Soc. Med.* 55: 311-16. Section of Psychiatry, pp. 1-6 (abridged).

1963

100. Slater, E. Diagnosis of zygosity by finger prints. *Acta Psychiat. Scand.* 39: 78-84.
101. Slater, E. Genetical factors in neurosis. *Proc. 2nd. Internat. Congr. Hum. Genet., (Rome, 1961),* pp. 1686-91. Rome: Istituto G. Mendel.
102. Slater, E. The colour imagery of poets. *Schweiz. Arch. Neurol. Neurochir. Psychiat.* 91: 303-8.
103. Cowie, V., and Slater, E. Maternal age and miscarriage in the mothers of mongols. *Acta Genet. (Basel)* 13: 77-83.
104. Slater, E., Beard, A. W., and Glithero, E. The schizophrenia-like psychoses of epilepsy. *Brit. J. Psychiat.* 109: 95-150.

1964

105. Slater, E. Genetical factors in neurosis. *Brit. J. Psychol.* 55: 265-69.
106. Slater, E. Review of *Psychogenic Psychoses* by P. M. Faergeman and *Die schizophrenie-ähnlichen Emotionspsychosen* by F. Labhardt. *Brit. J. Psychiat.* 110: 114-18.
107. Slater P., Shields J., and Slater, E. A quadratic discriminant of zygosity from fingerprints. *J. Med. Genet.* 1: 42-46.

1965

108. Slater, E. Clinical aspects of genetic mental disorders. In *Biochemical Aspects of Neurological Disorders* (2nd series), ed. J. N. Cumings and M. Kremer, pp. 271-85. Oxford: Blackwell.
109. Slater, E. Diagnosis of 'Hysteria'. *Brit. Med. J.* 1: 1395-99.
110. Slater, E. Discussion of paper by M. Bleuler, 'Conception of schizophrenia within the last fifty years and today'. *Internat. J. Psychiat.* 1: 318-19.
111. Slater, E. Obituary notice, F. J. Kallmann, *Brit. Med. J.* 1:1440.
112. Slater, E., and Glithero, E. A follow-up of patients diagnosed as suffering from 'Hysteria'. *J. Psychosom. Res.* 9: 9-13.
113. Coppen, A. J., Cowie, V. A., and Slater, E. Familial aspects of 'neuroticism' and 'extraversion'. *Brit. J. Psychiat.* 111: 70-83.

1966

114. Slater, E. Expectation of abnormality on paternal and maternal sides: a computational model. *J. Med. Genet.* 3: 159-61.
115. Slater, E. Pain and the psychiatrist. Letter in *Brit. J. Psychiat.* 112: 329.
116. Crome, L., Cowie, V. A., and Slater, E. A statistical note on cerebellar and brain-stem weight in mongolism. *J. Ment. Defic. Res.* 10: 69-72.
117. Shields, J., and Slater, E. La similarité du diagnostic chez les jumeaux et le problème de la spécificité biologique dans les névroses et les troubles de la personnalité [Diagnostic similarity in twins and the problem of biological specificity in the neuroses and personality disorders]. *Evolut. Psychiat.* 31: 441-51.
118. Slater, E. (unsigned). The genetics of schizophrenia. In *Medical Research Council Annual Report, April 1965-March 1966,* pp. 54-61. London: Her Majesty's Stationery Office.

1967

119. Slater, E. Distinguishing the effects of heredity and environment. Discussion of 'The psychogenesis of schizophrenia: a review of the literature' by Hans Kind. *Internat. J. Psychiat.* 3: 416-17.
120. Slater, E. Review of *On Aggression* by Konrad Lorenz. *Brit. J. Psychiat.* 113: 803-6.
121. Shields, J., and Slater, E. Genetic aspects of schizophrenia. *Hosp. Med. (Lond.)* 1: 579-84.

122. Slater, E. Genetics of criminals. *World Med. 2 (12):* 44-45.
123. Slater, E. Vote of thanks to Dr. A. H. Halsey on the occasion of the Galton Lecture 1967. Eugen. Rev. 59: 149.
124. Slater, E. Genetic factors and schizophrenia. Transcript of the Symposium on Biological Research in Schizophrenia (Moscow, November 28-December 2, 1967) ed. D. Lozovskii, pp. 109-13 (Russian) and 244-48 (English). Moscow: Akademia Meditsinskikh Nauk SSSR. Also in *Vestn. Acad. Med. Nauk SSSR (1969)* 4: 75-9 (in Russian).
125. Shields, J., Gottesman, I. I., and Slater, E. Kallmann's 1946 schizophrenic twin study in the light of new information. *Acta Psychiat. Scand.* 43: 385-96.

1968
126. Slater, E. Review of *ESP: A Scientific Evaluation* by C. E. M. Hansel. *Brit. J. Psychiat.* 114: 653-58.
127. Slater, E., and Tsuang, M-t. Abnormality on paternal and maternal sides: observations in schizophrenia and manic-depression. *J. Med. Genet.* 5: 197-99.
128. Slater, E. Mental disorders: genetic aspects. In *International Encyclopedia of the Social Sciences,* pp. 127-33. New York: Macmillan and Free Press.
129. Cowie, V. A., and Slater, E. The fertility of mothers of mongols. *J. Ment. Defic. Res.* 12: 196-208.
130. Cowie, J., Cowie, V. A., and Slater, E. *Delinquency in Girls.* London: Heinemann.
131. Slater, E. A review of earlier evidence on genetic factors in schizophrenia. In *The Transmission of Schizophrenia,* eds D. Rosenthal and S. S. Kety, pp. 15-26. Oxford: Pergamon. (Also issued as *J. Psychiat. Res.* 6: Suppl 1, 15-26.)
132. Slater, E. La herencia en las psicosis endogenas [Heredity in the endogenous psychoses], translated by César Pérez de Francisco. *Neurologiá-Neurocirugía Psiquiatria* 9: 137-49; and *Revistá Gharma* 34: 9-20 (1969).
133. Slater, E. *The Ebbless Sea, Poems 1922-1962.* London: Outposts Publications.
134. Slater, E. A note on terms of art in 'Hamlet'. *Shakespearean Authorship Review* 20: 1-4.

1969
135. Slater, E., and Shields, J. Genetical aspects of anxiety. In *Studies of Anxiety,* ed. M. H. Lader, pp. 62-71. *Brit. J. Psychiat.,* Special Publn. No. 3. Ashford (Kent): Headley.
136. Slater, E., and Moran, P. A. P. The schizophrenia-like psychoses of epilepsy: relation between ages of onset. *Brit. J. Psychiat.* 115: 599-600.
137. Slater, E., and Roth, M. *Mayer-Gross, Slater and Roth Clinical Psychiatry,* 3rd. ed. London: Baillière, Tindall and Cassell.
138. Slater, E. Choosing the time to die. In *Proceedings, 5th International Conference on Suicide Prevention,* London 1969, ed. R. Fox. pp. 269-72. Vienna: International Association for Suicide Prevention.
139. Slater, E. Death: the biological aspect. In *Euthanasia and the Right to Death. The Case for Voluntary Euthanasia,* ed. A. B. Downing, pp. 49-60. London: Peter Owen.
140. Slater, E. Review of *Genetic and Environmental Influences on Behaviour, Eugenics Society Symposium, Sept. 1967* ed. J. M. Thoday and A. S. Parkes. *J. Med. Genet* 6: 447-48.
141. Slater, E. Review of *Selected Topics in Medical Genetics* ed. C. A. Clarke. *J. Med Genet.* 6:444-45.
142. Slater, E. An anonymous contribution, to the section entitled 'Heredity and Environment', in *How to Adopt.* London: Consumers Association.

143. Slater, E. Review of *The Biological Time Bomb* by G. R. Taylor. *Brit. J. Psychiat.* 115:355.
144. Slater, E. A psychiatric view of Shakespeare's sonnets. *An. port. Psiquit.* 21: 545-72.

1970

145. Kahn, J., Carter, W. I., Dernley, N., and Slater, E. Chromosome studies in remand home and prison populations. In *Criminological Implications of Chromosome abnormalities,* ed. D. J. West. Cambridge: Institute of Criminology.
146. Slater, E. Review of *Death and Bereavement* ed. A. H. Kutscher, and of *Man's Concern with Death* by A. Toynbee *et al. Brit. J. Psychiat.* 116: 450.
147. Slater, E. Discussion of *The Families of Schizophrenic Patients* by Y. O. Alanen. *Proc. roy. Soc. Med.* 63: 230-31.
148. Slater, E. 'Chairman's Introduction', to Sex ratios in different populations. In *Biosocial Aspects of Sex* (Proceedings of the 6th Annual Symposium of the Eugenics Society, London, Sept. 1969). *J. Biosoc. Sci.* Suppl. 2, 53.
149. Slater, E. Review of *The Place of Dynamic Psychiatry in Medicine* by H. H. Wolff *Brit. J. Psychiat.* 117: 454.
150. Slater, E. The problems of pathography. In *Studies Dedicated to Erik Essen-Möller. Acta Psychiat. Scand.* Suppl. 219, pp. 209-15.
151. Slater, E. Attitudes to conservation. Letter in *Nature* 225: Feb 21, 773.
152. Slater, E. Review of *Tantalizers: A Book of Original Logical Puzzles* by Martin Hollis. *Brit. J. Psychiat.* 117: 603-04.
153. Slater, E. Review of *Mythopoiesis: Mythic Patterns in the Literary Classics* by H. Slochover. *Brit. J. Psychiat.* 117: 591.

1971

154. Slater, E., and Cowie, V. *The Genetics of Mental Disorders.* London: Oxford University Press.
155. Slater, E. Review of *Sanity, Madness and the Family: Families of Schizophrenics,* (2nd ed.) by R. D. Laing and A. Esterson. *Brit. J. Psychiat.* 118: 111-12.
156. Slater, E. Review of *Churchill: Four Faces and the Man* by A. J. P. Taylor, R. R. James, J. H. Plumb, B. L. Hart and A. Storr. *Brit. J. Psychiat.* 118: 98-99.
157. Slater, E. Review of *The Honest Politician's Guide to Crime Control* by N. Morris and G. Hawkins. *Brit. J. Psychiat.* 118: 102.
158. Slater, E. Review of *The Right to Abortion: a Psychiatric View* (formulated by the Committee on Psychiatry and Law Group for the Advancement of Psychiatry). *Brit. J. Psychiat.* 118:126.
159. Slater, E. Review of *The Biocrats* by G. Leach. *Brit. J. Psychiat.* 118: 361-62.
160. Slater, E., Maxwell, J., and Price, J. S. Distribution of ancestral secondary cases in bipolar affective disorders. *Brit. J. Psychiat.* 118: 215-18.
161. Slater, E. Review of *The Psychology of Suicide* by E. S. Shneidman, N. L. Farberow and R. E. Litman. *Brit. J. Psychiat.* 119:108-09.
162. Slater, E. Health Service or Sickness Service? *Brit. Med. J.* 4: 734-36.
163. Slater, E. Letter regarding paediatric cardiology. *Brit. Med. J.* 18 Sept, 702.
164. Slater, E. Science and non-science in psychiatry. Letter in *Lancet* 20 March, 599-600.
165. Slater, E. Review of *The Doomsday Book* by G. Rattray Taylor. *Brit. J. Psychiat.* 119: 334-35.
166. Slater, E., Hare, E. H., and Price, J. S. Marriage and fertility of psychiatric patients compared with national data. In *Differential Reproduction in Individuals with Mental and Physical Disorders,* (ed. I. I. Gottesman and L. Erlenmeyer-Kimling). *Social Biology* 18: Supplement, S. 60-S73.

167. Hare, E. H., Price, J. S., and Slater, E. T. O. The age-distribution of schizophrenia and neurosis: findings in a national sample. *Brit. J. Psychiat.* 119: 445-48.

168. Price, J. S., Slater, E., and Hare, E. H. Marital status of first admissions to psychiatric beds in England and Wales in 1965 and 1966. In *Differential Reproduction in Individuals with Mental and Physical Disorders,* (ed. I. I. Gottesman and L. Erlenmeyer-Kimling). *Social Biology* 18: Supplement, S74-S94.

169. Slater, E. *General Practitioner* Nov. 26, p. 21, 'Freud's ideas cannot lead to a science of the unconscious'.

170. Slater, E. *Autobiographical Sketch,* and *Retrospect.* In *Man, Mind and Heredity, Selected Papers of Eliot Slater on Psychiatry and Genetics,* eds. J. Shields and I. I. Gottesman, pp. 1-23 and 367-80. Baltimore: Johns Hopkins.

1972

171. Sargant, W. and Slater, E.. (assisted by D. Kelly) (1972). *An Introduction to Physical Methods of Treatment in Psychiatry,* 5th ed. Edinburgh and London: Churchill Livingstone.

172. Slater, E. The case for a major partially dominant gene. In *Genetic Factors in 'Schizophrenia',* ed. A. R. Kaplan. pp. 173-80. Springfield, Ill: Charles C. Thomas.

173. Slater, E. Priorities in health work. *Health Magazine* 9: 1 March, 22-23.

174. Hare, E. H., Price. J. S., and Slater, E. Letter 'Schizophrenia and season of birth'. In *Brit. J. Psychiat.* 120: 124-25.

175. Slater, E. Is psychiatry a science? Does it want to be? *World Medicine* Annual Review, Feb., pp. 79-81.

176. Slater, E. Review of *The Future of Man* eds. F. J. Ebling and G. W. Heath. *Eugenics Society Bulletin* 4: 2, June.

177. Hare, E. H., Price, J. S., and Slater, E. Fertility in obsessional neurosis. *Brit. J. Psychiat.* 121: 197-205.

178. Slater, E. General Introduction: Ethics and the population increase. In *Population and Pollution,* eds. Peter R. Cox and John Peel, pp 1-5. London: Academic Press.

179. Hare, E. H., Price, J. S. and Slater, E. Parental social class in psychiatric patients. *Brit. J. Psychiat.* 121: 515-24.

180. Slater, E. The psychiatrist in search of a science. I: Early thinkers at the Maudsley. *Brit. J. Psychiat.* 121: 591-98.

181. Slater, E. Resources and population. *Bulletin of the Eugenics Society* 4: December, 86-91.

182. Slater, E. Foreword. In *Schizophrenia and Genetics: a Twin Study Vantage Point,* by I. I. Gottesman and J. Shields, pp. xi-xiv. New York: Academic Press.

183. Slater, E. The illness of Rudolf Hess. A phenomenological analysis. In *Dimensiones de la Psiquiatria Contemporanea,* pp. 191-210. ed. C. P. de Francisco. Mexico: Editorial Fournia, S. A.

1973

184. Slater, E. New horizons in medical ethics: severely malformed children. *Brit. Med. J.* 2: 284-89.

185. Slater, E. A statistical note on 'A Lover's Complaint'. *Notes and Queries* New Series, 20: 4, 138-40.

186. Slater, E. The psychiatrist in search of a science: II. Developments in the logic and the sociology of science. *Brit. J. Psychiat.* 122: 625-36.

187. Slater, E. Review of *Jung* by A. Storr. *Brit. J. Psychiat.* 123: 364-65.

188. Spicer, C. C., Hare, E. H., and Slater, E. Neurotic and psychotic forms of depressive illness: evidence from age-incidence in a national sample. *Brit. J. Psychiat.* 123: 535-41.

189. Slater, E. Race, sex and equality. *New Statesman* 6 April, 491-93.
190. Hare, E. H., Price, J. S. and Slater, E. Mental disorder and season of birth. *Nature* 241:480.
191. Slater, E. Review of *The Stranger in Shakespeare* by L. A. Fiedler. *Brit. J. Psychiat.* 124:312.
192. Slater, E. Sex and equality. *Women Speaking* Oct-Dec., 4-6.

1974
193. Hare, E. H., Price, J. S., and Slater, E. Mental disorder and season of birth: a national sample compared with the general population. *Brit. J. Psychiat.* 124: 81-86.
194. Slater, E. Wandlung der ethischen Auffassung über Euthanasie in England [The changing ethical view of euthanasia in England, translated by Ingrid Veitinger]. In *Alter und Tod—annehmen oder verdrangen? Conference Report,* ed. W. Bitter. pp. 139-46. Stuttgart: Ernst Klett.
195. Slater, E. New Biology—New Ethics. In *Population and the New Biology. Proceedings of the 10th Annual Symposium of the Eugenics Society, London, 1973,* ed. B. Benjamin, P. R. Cox and J. Peel, pp. 177-80. London and New York: Academic Press.
196. Slater, E. Foreword. In *Biological Mechanisms of Schizophrenia and Schizophrenia-like Psychoses,* pp. v-vi, ed H. Mitsuda and T. Fukuda. Tokyo: Igaku Shoin.
197. Slater, E. Early thinkers at the Maudsley (the first of the three papers). Reprinted in *Institute of Psychiatry 1924-1974,* pp. 64-69. London: Institute of Psychiatry.

1975
198. Slater, E. Review of *Awakenings* by O. Sacks. *Brit. J. Psychiat.* 126: 92-93.
199. Shields, J. and Slater, E. Genetic aspects of schizophrenia. In *Contemporary Psychiatry,* ed. T. Silverstone and B. Barraclough, pp. 32-40. Brit. J. Psychiat. Special Publn. No. 9. Ashford, Kent: Headley.
200. Slater, E. Foreword. In *Contemporary Psychiatry,* ed. T. Silverstone and B. Barraclough, pp. xiii-xv. *Brit. J. Psychiat* Special Publn. No. 9. Ashford, Kent: Headley.
201. Slater, E. Psychiatry in the 'thirties'. *Contemporary Review* 226: 70-75.
202. Slater, E. The psychiatrist in search of a science: III. The Depth Psychologies. *Brit. J. Psychiat.* 126: 205-24.
203. Slater, E. Word links with 'The Merry Wives of Windsor'. *Notes and Queries.* April 169-71.
204. Slater, E. Shakespeare: word links between poems and plays. *Notes and Queries.* April 157-163.
205. Slater, E. Some psychological aspects of the Sonnets. *The Bard* 1: 1-8.
206. Slater, E. Psychiatry in the thirties. *Bethlem and Maudsley Gazette* Spring 8-10. (Reprinted from *Contemporary Review,* see 202 above.)
207. Slater, E. Review of *Creative Malady: Illness in the Lives and Minds of Charles Darwin, Florence Nightingale, Mary Baker Eddy, Sigmund Freud, Marcel Proust, Elizabeth Barrett Browning* by George Pickering. *Brit. J. Psychiat.* 127:93.
208. Slater, E. Review of *Genetic Research in Psychiatry* eds. R. R. Fieve, D. Rosenthal and H. Brill. *New Psychiatry* Oct. 23, 18-19.
209. Slater, E. The ordeal of Evelyn Waugh. Review of *Evelyn Waugh: A Biography* by C. Sykes *Brit. Med. J.* 13 Dec.

1976
210. Slater, E. What is hysteria? *New Psychiatry* 3: 714-15.
211. Slater, E. Sinne of Self-love. *Notes and Queries* April 155-56.

212. Slater, E., Flew, A. G. M. and Downing, A. B. *Death with Dignity*. London: The Voluntary Euthanasia Society.
213. Slater, E. Review of *Francis Galton: The Life and Work of a Victorian Genius* by D. W. Forrest. *J. Biosoc. Sci.* 8: 75-77.
214. Slater, E. Assisted suicide: some ethical considerations. *Internat. J. Health Services* 6: 2, 321-30.
215. Slater, E. In search of courage. *World Medicine* 11: 51 and 53.
216. Slater, E. Eugenics. In *Encyclopaedic Handbook of Medical Psychology,* ed. Stephen Krauss, pp. 181-86. London: Butterworths.
217. Slater, E. A reading of 'Sonnet 120'. *The Bard* 1: 2, 43-46.
218. Slater, E. Review of *Psychopath: The case of Patrick Mackay* by T. Clark and J. Penycate and *The Social Psychology of Mental Disorder* by J. Orford. *New Statesman* 10 Dec., 842-44.
219. Slater, E. Altruistic suicide. *Catholic Medical Quarterly* 27: 4, 197-201.

1977

220. Slater, E. Word Links with 'All's Well that Ends Well'. *Notes and Queries* 24: 109-12.
221. Slater, E. Review of *The Diaries of Evelyn Waugh* ed. M. Davies. *Brit. J. Psychiat.* 31: 320.
222. Slater, E. Review of *Superminds: An Investigation into the Paranormal* by John Taylor. *Notes and Queries* July-Aug., 384.
223. Slater, E. Eugenics 1900-1914. Review of *Eugenics and Politics in Britain 1900-1914* by G. R. Searle. *The Eugenics Society Bulletin* 9: 4, 128-31.
224. Slater, E. Biological differences and social justice [E. S. Vickers Lecture]. In *Developments in Psychiatric Research,* ed. J. M. Tanner 199-212. London: Hodder & Stoughton.
225. Slater, E. How dottissima? Review of *Marie Stopes* by Ruth Hall. *The New Review,* 4, 44, 52-53.
226. Slater, E. Qui sont les bienfaiteurs? *L'Evolution Psychiatrique* XLII: 1047-53. (A revised version of unpublished paper, The social value of an elite, read at the symposium Human Differences and Social Issues, London, August 1970).
227. Slater, E., and Roth, M. *Mayer-Gross, Slater and Roth Clinical Psychiatry,* revised reprint of 3rd ed. London: Baillière Tindall.
228. Slater, E. Review of *Homosexuality and Literature 1890–1930* by Jeffrey Meyers. *Notes and Queries* April 181-82.

1978

229. Slater, E. Gone and future. Review of *1975 (1984 minus 9),* by Hans Keller. *The New Review* 45/6.
230. Slater, E. Word links between 'Timon of Athens' and 'King Lear'. *Notes and Queries* April 147-49.
231. Slater, E. Review of *Memory and Mind* by Norman Malcolm. *Notes and Queries* June 285-86.
232. Slater, E. Obituary for James Shields. *Nature* 274: 728-29.
233. Slater, E. Review of *Russia's Political Hospitals. The Abuse of Psychiatry in the Soviet Union* by S. Bloch and P. Reddaway, *Journal of Medical Ethics* 4: 100-03.
234. Slater, E. On accepting the Second Annual Theodosius Dobzhansky Memorial Award for research in behaviour genetics. *Behaviour Genetics* 8:6, 533-34.
235. Slater, E. Word links from 'Troilus' to 'Othello' and 'Macbeth'. *The Bard* 2: 4-22.